Diabetes
COOKBOOK

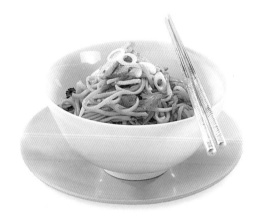

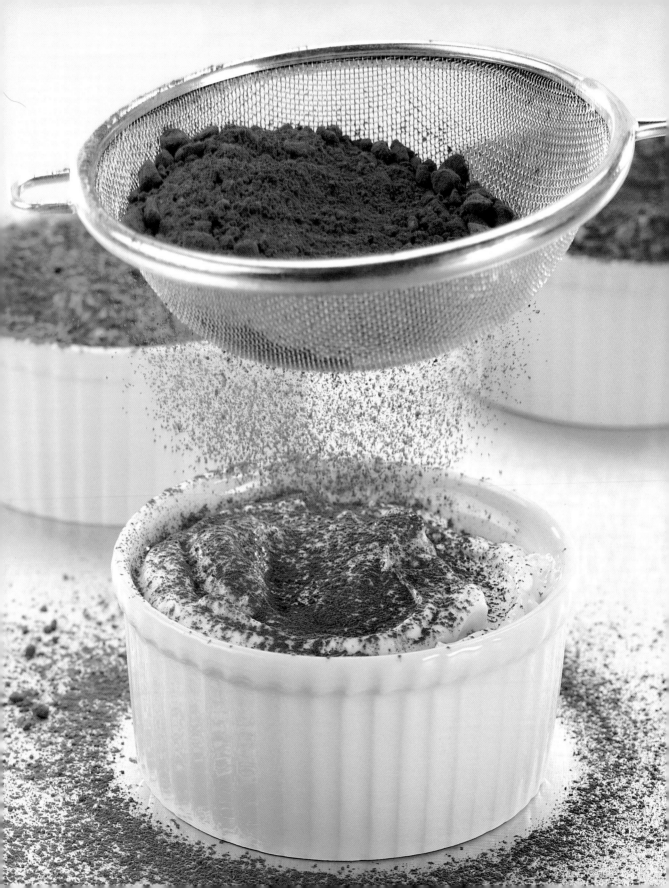

IN ASSOCIATION WITH
THE AMERICAN DIABETES ASSOCIATION

Diabetes
COOKBOOK

PHOTOGRAPHY SIMON SMITH

FOOD STYLING SALLY MANSFIELD

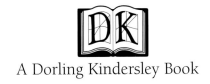

A Dorling Kindersley Book

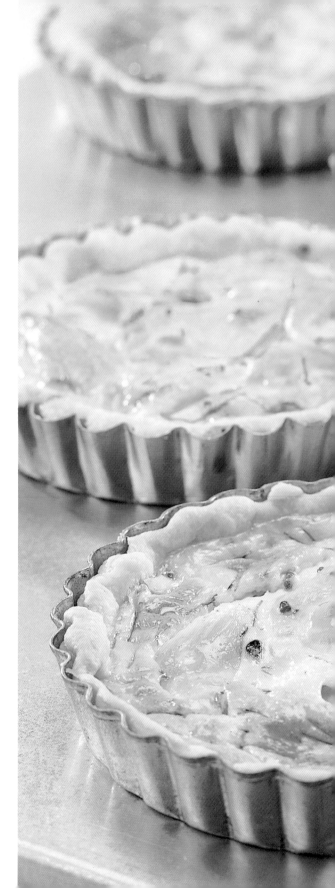

Dorling 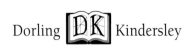 Kindersley

LONDON, NEW YORK, MUNICH, MELBOURNE AND DELHI

Text produced by Diabetes UK
Recipes Louise Tyler
Diabetes & the Diet Lyndel Costain

Editor Janice Anderson
Art Editor Toni Kay
US Editors Barbara Minton, Tracy McCord
Senior Managing Editor Krystyna Mayer
Deputy Art Director Carole Ash
DTP Designer Conrad van Dyk
Production Controller Joanna Bull

Published in the United States by
Dorling Kindersley Publishing Inc.
375 Hudson Street
New York, New York 10014

8 10 9

ISBN 0-7894-5175-1.   00-027079

Reproduced in Italy by GRB Editrice, Verona
Printed and bound in China by L.Rex Printing Co. Ltd

Recipe Points to Remember
Spoon measurements are level, unless otherwise
stated. Eggs are medium, unless otherwise stated.
Follow either metric or imperial measurements,
never mix the two. Baking times are a guide
only, because every oven varies.

Discover more at
www.dk.com

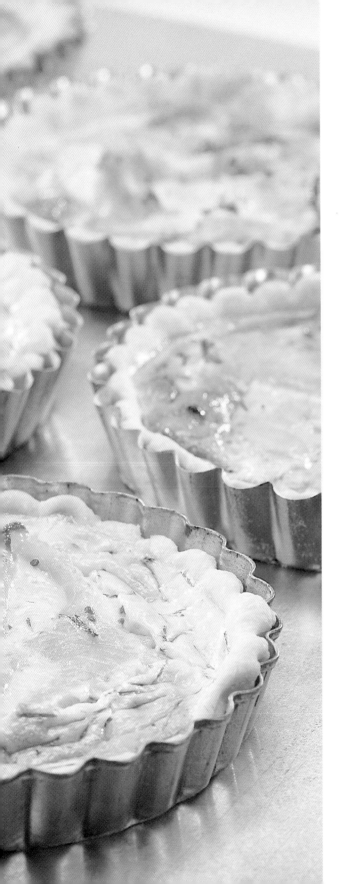

Contents

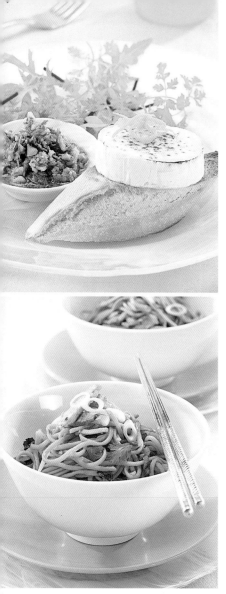

FOREWORD

Almost 16 million Americans have diabetes, about 6 percent of the US population. In 1999, it was estimated that 500,000 to 1 million people had Type 1 diabetes, and another 9.5 million people have been diagnosed with Type 2. Whichever type you have, food is probably a big problem in your life.

Being diagnosed with diabetes often means that you need to change your eating habits. The millions of us who have ever tried a "diet" know exactly how hard it is to change how and what we eat. That's why the American Diabetes Association has teamed up with Dorling Kindersley Publishing to offer this appealing cookbook with recipes that are both healthy and tasty.

The American Diabetes Association is the nation's leading voluntary health organization supporting diabetes research, information, and advocacy. Founded in 1940, the Association provides services to communities across the country. Its mission is to prevent and cure diabetes and to improve the lives of all people affected by diabetes.

For more than 50 years, the American Diabetes Association has been the leading publisher of comprehensive diabetes information for people with diabetes and the health care professionals that treat them. Its huge library of practical and authoritative books for people with diabetes covers every aspect of living with the disease – cooking and nutrition, fitness, weight control, medications, complications, emotional issues, and general self-care. Membership in the Association is available to everyone and includes a subscription to *Diabetes Forecast*, the nation's leading health and wellness magazine for people with diabetes.

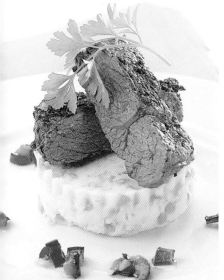

American Diabetes Association

INTRODUCTION

Diet plays a major role in controlling diabetes and reducing the risk of developing complications. This book is both a superb cookbook and a complete guide to food based on the dietary recommendations for diabetes. The recipes are low in fat, salt, and sugar and are based on a variety of starchy staple foods, fresh fruits and vegetables, and the right kinds of fat. Each recipe has a nutritional analysis to help in balancing food choices and maintaining a healthy diet.

There is no such thing as a single diet suitable for everyone with diabetes. An individual's dietary requirements are dependent on many factors, including age, build, whether he or she is overweight or underweight, and levels of physical activity. Anyone newly diagnosed with diabetes should see a qualified dietitian for advice specific to the individual's dietary needs.

Whatever type of diabetes a person has, the right eating habits help control blood glucose levels, weight, lipid or fat levels, and other aspects of diabetes. Dietary priorities will change over time, particularly if diabetes is diagnosed in childhood, when growth requirements are most important and when regular review is essential. Many people with Type 2 diabetes, the most common type, are overweight; for this group, losing weight is the priority. The aim of all dietary advice is to make life easier, through simple changes that can be maintained over the long-term rather than by radical changes that cannot. Although people with diabetes should limit high-fat, high-sugar foods in their diet, it is possible to balance choices and enjoy a wide variety of foods. The important thing to remember about healthy eating when you have diabetes is to make changes to your eating habits and food choices that you can maintain and that will help you manage your diabetes more easily.

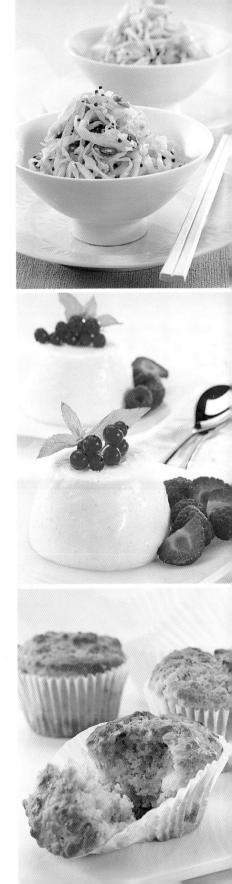

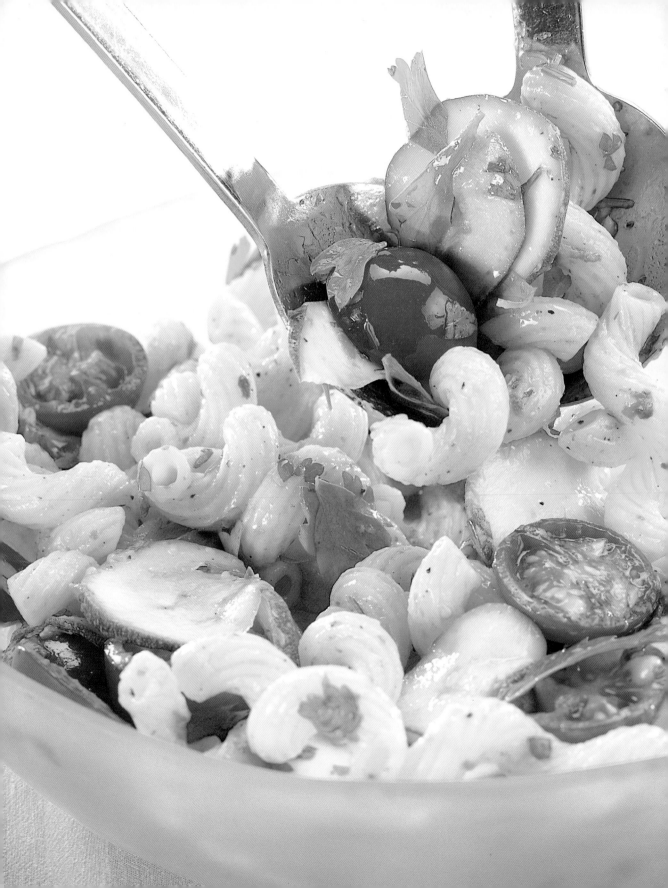

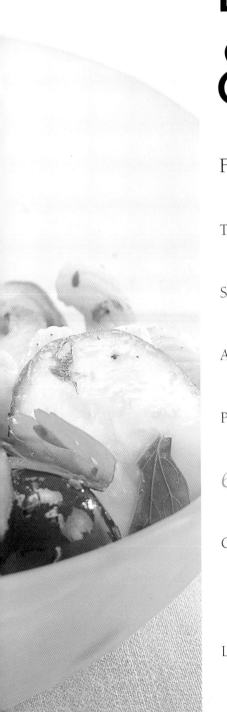

DIABETES & THE DIET

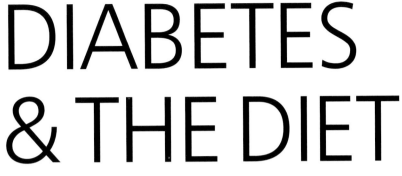

FOR PEOPLE WHO HAVE DIABETES, FOLLOWING A DIET THAT IS *right for them* IS ESSENTIAL. THIS SECTION OF THE BOOK IS *a guide* TO HOW SUCH A DIET CAN BE *achieved.* ITS GOAL IS TO HELP PEOPLE TO MAKE REALISTIC ADJUSTMENTS TO *eating habits* AND *food choices* THAT CAN BE MANAGED ON A LONG-TERM BASIS.

LEFT: HERBED PASTA SALAD *(see page 81)*

UNDERSTANDING DIABETES

DIABETES IS A CONDITION WHERE THERE IS TOO MUCH GLUCOSE IN THE BLOOD. IT DEVELOPS
BECAUSE OF A LACK OF, OR A PROBLEM WITH THE USE, OF INSULIN, A HORMONE THAT IS PRODUCED
BY THE PANCREAS. INSULIN CONTROLS THE BODY'S BLOOD GLUCOSE LEVELS BY ALLOWING
GLUCOSE TO ENTER BODY CELLS, WHERE IT IS USED AS ENERGY-GIVING FUEL.

**THE MAIN SYMPTOMS
OF UNTREATED DIABETES**

○ Thirst and a dry mouth

○ Passing large amounts
of urine (especially
during the night)

○ Fatigue

○ Weight loss

○ Blurred vision

GLOBAL STATISTICS

Worldwide, diabetes is on
the increase. Currently,
2.1 percent of the world's
population, or 124 million
people, has diabetes. In the
US there are an estimated
16 million people with
diabetes. Diabetes is more
common among certain
ethnic groups. In Asia and
Africa, diabetes could
become two to three times
more common in 2010
than it is today.

Insulin and glucose

When glucose is unable to get into cells properly, too much is left in the blood, and the body does not get the fuel it needs to stay healthy. The liver makes glucose and passes it into the blood stream, but glucose in the blood comes mainly from the digestion of carbohydrate-rich foods. These can be starchy foods like potatoes, bread, and pasta; or sugary foods and drinks. So if, after a meal, the body does not produce enough insulin, blood glucose levels rise and stay high. High glucose levels cause fatigue and thirst, and the passing of large amounts of urine. There may also be blurred vision. These are all common symptoms of untreated diabetes (*see box, left*).

THE TWO MAIN TYPES OF DIABETES

Type 1 (insulin dependent) develops when the body produces little or no insulin. It affects people under 40 years of age and is treated by a combination of insulin injections and a healthy, balanced diet based on regular meals and snacks.

Type 2 (noninsulin dependent) is the most common type of diabetes and develops when the body can still make its own insulin, but not enough for its needs, or when the insulin that the body does make is not used properly. Type 2 diabetes usually affects people over 40 years of age, and is treated by diet alone, or diet and tablets, or by a combination of diet and insulin.

Diabetes world-wide

Diabetes is a common condition, affecting over 2 percent of the adult population in many developed countries. It is estimated that for every person who has been diagnosed, there is another walking around undiagnosed and, therefore, untreated. Type 2 diabetes is more common than Type 1 diabetes.

The causes of diabetes

There is no single cause of diabetes and a combination of both genetic (diabetes tends to run in families) and environmental factors appear to lie behind it. In addition, scientists are still not exactly sure what causes the pancreas to stop producing enough insulin. It may be that a virus or the body's own immune system destroys the insulin-producing cells of the pancreas. Type 2 diabetes is also linked to obesity, especially when there is excess weight around the stomach. As obesity increases worldwide, so does Type 2 diabetes.

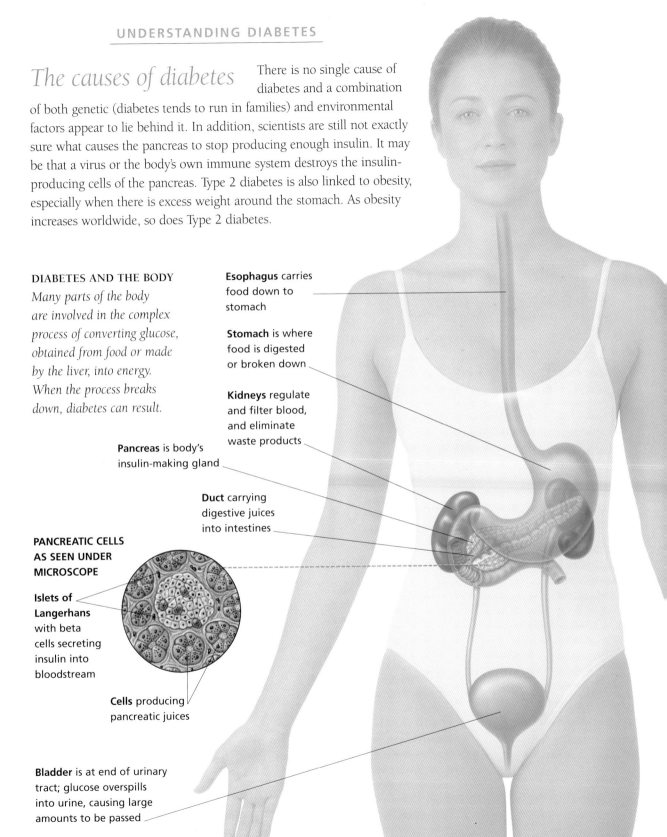

DIABETES AND THE BODY
Many parts of the body are involved in the complex process of converting glucose, obtained from food or made by the liver, into energy. When the process breaks down, diabetes can result.

Esophagus carries food down to stomach

Stomach is where food is digested or broken down

Kidneys regulate and filter blood, and eliminate waste products

Pancreas is body's insulin-making gland

Duct carrying digestive juices into intestines

PANCREATIC CELLS AS SEEN UNDER MICROSCOPE

Islets of Langerhans with beta cells secreting insulin into bloodstream

Cells producing pancreatic juices

Bladder is at end of urinary tract; glucose overspills into urine, causing large amounts to be passed

CONTROLLING DIABETES

THE MAIN AIM OF TREATMENT FOR ALL TYPES OF DIABETES IS TO CONTROL GLUCOSE LEVELS

AND REDUCE THE RISK OF DEVELOPING THE LONG-TERM COMPLICATIONS LINKED TO THE CONDITION,

SUCH AS EYE AND KIDNEY PROBLEMS, CORONARY HEART DISEASE (CHD), AND NERVE DAMAGE.

Checking up

It is really important that you have regular medical checkups. Your doctor or the local hospital can look out for warning signs of any health problems, such as high cholesterol (people with diabetes have four times the risk of developing CHD than people without), high levels of triglycerides, (another type of fat in the blood that is linked to CHD), high blood pressure, cataracts, or nerve complications. Your doctor or hospital staff will also provide ongoing information and support to help you manage your diabetes, including referral to other health professionals in your area, such as qualified dietitians.

Controlling weight

Weight control is an essential part of managing diabetes. Use the chart on the right to assess your weight. If it indicates that you need to lose weight, be realistic and aim to lose weight gradually – say 2–3lb per month. Keep a food diary to learn more about your eating habits, and use it to make step-by-step changes. Do not go it alone – enlist support from family, friends, a health professional, or weight watching groups.

BODY MASS INDEX CHART

This chart applies to both men and women. To assess your weight, take a straight line across from your height (without shoes) and a line up from your weight (without clothes). Put a mark where the two lines meet.

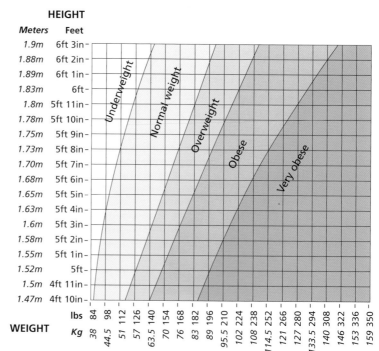

KEY TO CHART

Underweight You may need to eat more. Go for well-balanced, nutritious foods, rather than fatty snacks.

Normal weight You are eating the right quantity of food. Be sure you get a healthy balance in your diet.

Overweight You should try to lose some weight.

Obese You need to lose weight.

Very obese You urgently need to lose weight. See your doctor, who may refer you to a dietitian.

Reducing risks

Enjoying a healthy, balanced diet and, if needed, taking insulin injections or pills, will reduce the risk of complications. You should also:

● **Get to and keep at a healthy weight** (*see opposite*). Being at a healthy weight will help your body to use insulin more effectively.

● **Be physically active every day.** Any activity is of benefit, so choose something you enjoy doing. If possible, aim to be moderately active and undertake brisk walking, cycling, swimming, dancing, or gardening, for 30 minutes, five times a week.

● **If you smoke, plan to stop.** Smoking greatly increases your risk of getting lung cancer, and also further increases your risk of CHD and of stroke. Smoking is also a risk factor in the development of osteoporosis.

● **Drink alcohol in moderation** and keep to healthy limits (*see page 15*). You should never drink on an empty stomach since alcohol taken without food can make hypoglycemia (*see below*) more likely to occur.

● **Find time for relaxation,** especially if you frequently feel stressed.

HYPOGLYCEMIA

HYPOGLYCEMIA IS THE MEDICAL TERM FOR A LOW GLUCOSE LEVEL. AS GLUCOSE

IS AN ESSENTIAL FUEL FOR THE BODY, A BIG DROP IN ITS LEVEL CAN RAPIDLY MAKE YOU FEEL

UNWELL. THERE ARE A NUMBER OF REASONS WHY A HYPOGLYCEMIC EPISODE MAY OCCUR,

NO MATTER HOW GOOD YOUR CONTROL OF YOUR DIABETES IS.

Causes

The most common cause of a hypoglycemic episode is missing a snack or a meal or having too little carbohydrate at a meal. Occasionally, it can be caused by unplanned exercise, an imbalance in your insulin or pill dose, or drinking alcohol without food. Balancing food, exercise, and insulin, combined with regular blood glucose monitoring, is the key to avoiding a hypoglycemic epidose. Even with good control of your diabetes, though, you cannot predict everything that may happen.

Treatment

Rapid treatment, as soon as you recognize any symptoms (*see right*), is essential. Take a "short" or "quick-acting" carbohydrate, such as a glass of fruit juice or non-diet soft drink; two to five glucose tablets; one packet of glucose gel; or a small chocolate bar. To prevent glucose levels from dropping again, follow this with a "longer acting", starchy carbohydrate: a sandwich; a roll with peanut butter; a bowl of cereal; a cereal bar plus fruit, or your next meal if it is due.

THE MAIN SYMPTOMS OF HYPOGLYCEMIA
○ Trembling
○ Tingling of the lips
○ Feeling hungry
○ Sweating
○ Paleness
○ Anxiety
○ Irritability
○ Difficulty in concentrating
○ Fast pulse and palpitations

EATING HEALTHILY

THERE IS NO SUCH THING AS A SPECIAL "DIABETIC DIET" THAT FITS EVERYONE. EACH INDIVIDUAL'S AGE, WEIGHT, ACTIVITY LEVELS, FOOD PREFERENCES, GENERAL HEALTH, MEDICATIONS TAKEN, AND LIFESTYLE MUST ALL BE CONSIDERED WHEN PLANNING A DIET. IT IS THEREFORE IMPORTANT THAT ANYONE NEWLY DIAGNOSED WITH DIABETES OBTAINS ADVICE FROM A QUALIFIED DIETITIAN.

SPECIAL DIETARY NEEDS

Two groups of people have particular needs.

Children

Children with diabetes need to eat regular meals and snacks to help control their blood glucose levels. Parents and teachers must bear in mind that children may forget to eat and are more spontaneously physically active than adults. As children are constantly growing, developing, and changing their lifestyles, regular dietary reviews by qualified dietitians as part of their ongoing care are essential to ensure that their changing nutritional needs are met.

Special Diets

Adults following special diets because of medical conditions, such as food allergy or celiac disease, should seek professional dietetic advice to ensure that their diets are suitable for diabetes and are balanced.

Why diet is important

Whatever type of diabetes you have, the foods you choose and your eating habits can help you to control your blood glucose levels. Diabetes is a lifelong condition, so establishing good eating habits that you can keep to in the long term is essential. Eating healthily can also positively influence other diabetes-related aspects of your health, such as your weight, blood pressure, and cholesterol and triglyceride levels. While taking these factors into consideration, bear in mind that a main function of food is to give pleasure. There is no reason why you should not enjoy food as much as anyone else. Diet for diabetes is not about eating diet foods or following complicated and restrictive meal plans. It is about enjoying a healthy balance of a wide variety of foods to suit your individual needs. In fact, the basic principles of a diet for diabetes are the same as the healthy eating recommendations for everyone.

Making changes

Six points for healthy eating are set out on the opposite page. Consider how your current diet compares to them, and whether you need to make changes. If you decide that you do, set yourself small targets or goals that you can use to assess your progress. Start by choosing foods that you feel you will be able to eat most easily or enjoy most. For example, an initial target could be switching from heavy cream to skim milk, or using a low-fat spread instead of butter. Another target could be to stop adding sugar to tea or coffee, or to use sugar-free drinks in place of ordinary ones. You may need to take more care to spread your food intake evenly over the day, making sure that you eat regular meals based on starchy foods like bread, pasta, and rice. Making small, manageable changes like these one at a time will make it easier to keep to the correct diet in the long term. For more detailed information about choosing foods, refer to Facts About Food (*pages 16–19*).

Six ways to healthy eating

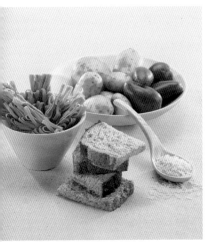

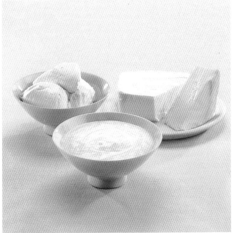

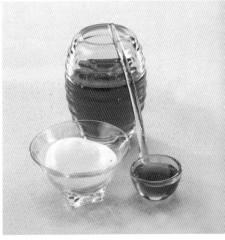

Eat regular meals based on starchy foods such as breads, pasta, potatoes, rice, noodles, and cereals. This will help to control glucose levels.

Cut down on fatty foods, replacing heavy cream and cheeses with lower fat foods such as low fat cream cheese, yogurt, and crème fraîche.

Put a limit on sugar and sugary foods. Having sugary drinks and too many sugary foods can make glucose rise too quickly.

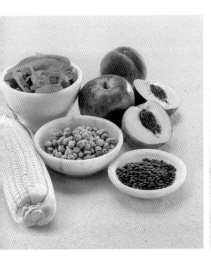

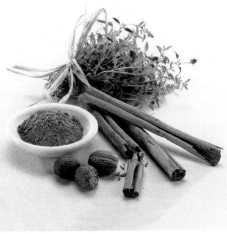

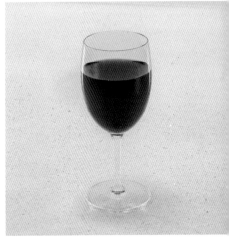

Eat more vegetables, fruits and legumes – at least five portions each day. See page 18 for some suggestions for foods that are appropriate portions.

Eat less salt and salty foods. Try flavoring foods with herbs and spices and look for reduced-salt prepared foods in cans and packages.

Drink alcohol in moderation. Have no more than 2 standard-measure drinks per day, if a man, and 1 if a woman. Try having a day or 2 a week without alcohol.

FACTS ABOUT FOOD

FOOD CHOICE AND EATING HABITS ARE IMPORTANT FACTORS IN HELPING PEOPLE WITH DIABETES
TO MANAGE THEIR CONDITION. THE HEALTHY DIET FOR A PERSON WITH DIABETES IS THE SAME
AS THE DIET RECOMMENDED FOR EVERYONE ELSE – LOW IN FAT, SALT, AND SUGAR, AND WITH
MEALS BASED ON STARCHY FOODS AND PLENTY OF FRUITS AND VEGETABLES.

A BALANCED PLATEFUL

*The ideal main course plate
for a person with diabetes
looks like this: half the plate
holds starchy food (here,
potatoes), two-thirds of the
other half of the plate holds
vegetables (or fruits), and
the remaining third holds
protein food, such as fish.*

Starchy foods

Starchy foods, including breads, cereals,
rice, pasta, noodles, and potatoes, are rich in
carbohydrate and are a healthy and naturally low fat source of fuel for
the body. The carbohydrate in starchy foods is digested to form glucose,
which is then absorbed into the blood. Most starchy foods are digested
and absorbed fairly slowly, leading to a gradual rise in blood sugar after
a meal or snack. Basing meals and snacks on starchy foods helps to
control glucose levels and even out the highs and lows.

● Baked potatoes and wholegrain starchy foods are also good sources
of fiber, which helps to prevent constipation and other bowel problems.

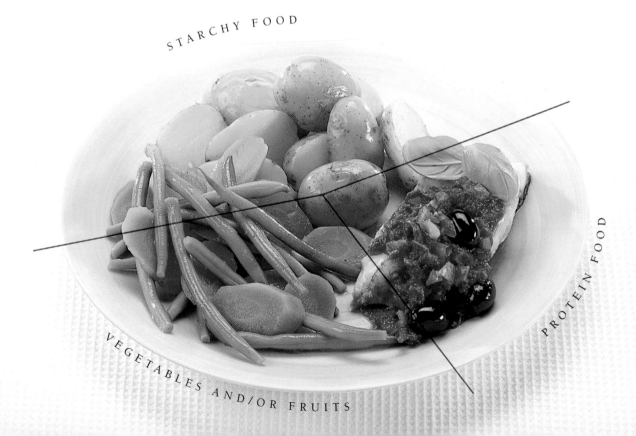

STARCHY FOOD

PROTEIN FOOD

VEGETABLES AND/OR FRUITS

- Some starchy foods are absorbed much more slowly and cause a more gradual rise in glucose levels than others. They have what is called a low Glycemic Index, or GI (*see box, right*). Foods like oatmeal, peas, beans, lentils, pasta, rye bread, apples, and oranges have low GIs. Interestingly, potatoes, cornflakes, rice, and white and wholewheat breads all have significantly higher GIs than these foods (but nowhere near as high as that of glucose).

- Making foods with a low GI a regular part of your meals may aid your glucose control by helping you to avoid "highs and lows". Although potatoes have a relatively high GI compared to foods like pasta, both potatoes and pasta are good choices: including a low-GI food like a bean salad, dhal, or baked beans in a potato meal reduces its overall GI level to that of a pasta meal

Sugar and sugary foods

A myth that continues to surround diabetes is that you must follow a sugar-free diet. It arose from the belief that all sugary foods caused a sudden and rapid rise in blood glucose levels. But the effect that any food or drink has on blood glucose levels depends not only on how much sugar it contains but also on a whole range of other factors, including the way it is cooked, how it is prepared, and what it is eaten with. A sugary drink taken on an empty stomach is absorbed quickly and raises blood glucose levels rapidly. However, sugar eaten as part of a meal will not raise blood sugar in the same way because it will be more slowly digested and absorbed (especially if the meal contains low-GI foods). For a healthy diet, limiting sugar is recommended for everyone.

Sweeteners

Artificial sweeteners made from aspartame, saccharin, acesulfame K, or cyclamate are sugar- and calorie-free and do not affect glucose levels. Artificial sweeteners can be used to sweeten foods after cooking or in recipes that do not need to be cooked (they can taste bitter or lose their sweetness if heated to high temperatures). They cannot, however, be used to replace sugar in baking. Sweeteners are classified as food additives, which means that they have been safety tested and approved for use in food processing. If, like many people with diabetes, you are regularly using sweeteners, try to choose products containing a variety of different types (check labels to see which sweetener has been used). If you are pregnant, you should discuss with your doctor the use of artificial sweeteners altogether.

GLYCEMIC INDEX

The Glycemic Index (GI) is a ranking of the measured effects of a wide range of carbohydrate-rich foods on blood glucose levels. Glucose is taken as the reference food, and its GI is 100 (the highest number on the Index), because it is the most rapidly absorbed of all carbohydrates and causes a sharp rise in glucose levels. The concept of GI can help people with diabetes to manage blood glucose levels more easily. The simplest application of GI is to combine starchy food with fruits, vegetables, and legumes. The idea is *not* to focus on individual indexes, but to apply the concept of GI in its most basic way.

BULK SWEETENERS

Bulk sweeteners, such as sorbitol, lacitol, and xylitol, which are carbohydrates, not sugars, and fructose, are approved for use in food processing in the US. They offer no special benefit over ordinary sugar and sweet foods.

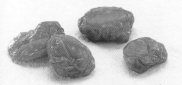

1 tablespoon of dried fruits

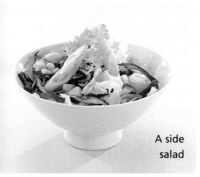

A side
salad

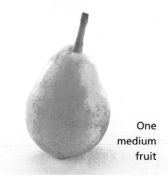

One
medium
fruit

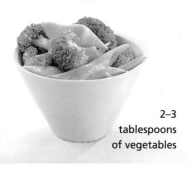

2–3
tablespoons
of vegetables

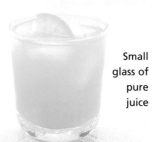

Small
glass of
pure
juice

Fruits and vegetables

A basic dietary recommendation for everyone is to eat at least five portions of fruits and vegetables every day (*see examples, left*). People who have diabetes can eat any type of fruit or vegetable, and should try to include some – fresh, frozen, canned, dried, or as pure juice – in most of their meals and snacks.

● Studies conducted in many countries have shown that people whose diets are rich in fruits and vegetables have a lower risk of developing a number of the world's chronic diseases, including CHD, stroke, and cancer.

● Fruits and vegetables are low in fat and calories, provide both soluble and insoluble fiber, are a good source of carbohydrate, and supply a broad range of vitamins, minerals, and phytochemicals (plant chemicals). The best known types of phytochemical are antioxidants – active compounds that help to neutralize potentially harmful free radicals in the body. Different fruits and vegetables provide different types of phytochemical, and eating a wide variety of them seems to be the best for our health. Vitamin supplements alone are no replacement for a diet rich in fruits and vegetables.

Fats

There are four main types of fat and no food or oil contains just one type of fatty acid (FA), the organic acids that make up fats and oils, but a mixture. While fats vary according to the type of fatty acid they contain, all fats are high in calories.

● **Saturates (SFAs)** Eating too many causes the liver to make more cholesterol. This can raise cholesterol levels, which in turn are linked to CHD. SFAs can also increase a tendency for blood to be more sticky, and so likely to clot. Cut down on SFAs.

● **Monounsaturates (MUFAs)** In moderation, these have beneficial effects on cholesterol levels, especially if used in place of saturates. Oils and spreads rich in MUFAs are recommended in preference to those rich in polyunsaturates (*see below*).

● **Polyunsaturates (PUFAs)** These have both a structural and a regulatory role. Some PUFAs are essential (EFAs) and there are two families: omega 6 and omega 3. These are needed for growth, the structure of cell membranes, and to produce "eicosanoids", chemical messengers that help to regulate functions such as blood clotting, blood pressure, and immunity. Omega 3 derivatives are also essential for early eye and brain development. As we usually get plenty of omega 6 FAs in our diets, particularly from margarines and spreads, we should limit these and consume more omega 3 FAs, for instance by eating oily fish, such as salmon, mackerel, sardines, pilchards, or trout, once a week. Fish oils are another good source of omega 3 FAs.

● **Trans Fatty Acids (TFAs)** Most of these are by-products of a process called hydrogenation, which makes unsaturated fatty acids firmer. Studies have shown than TFAs, like SFAs, can raise cholesterol levels, so they should be limited. Any food that has "hydrogenated vegetable oil/fats" high up in the ingredients list will contain significant amounts of TFAs. The most significant sources of TFAs are manufactured foods, such as cookies, pastries, and cakes.

Salt A high salt diet is linked to high blood pressure, CHD, stroke, and kidney problems, all potential long-term complications of diabetes. Around three-quarters of the salt we eat comes from processed foods, the rest from salt added during cooking and at the table. Try to limit using processed foods and ready-made meals; instead, cook your own meals, so that you can control how much salt goes into your food. Use herbs, spices, garlic, lemon juice, vinegars, and tomato paste to add flavor to dishes in place of salt. The amount of salt we consume tends to be linked to habit.

Fiber Everyone should enjoy a wide variety of fiber-rich foods as part of a healthy, balanced diet. Most fiber-rich foods are naturally low in fat, are a source of carbohydrate, and contain plenty of vitamins, minerals, and antioxidants. There are two main types:

● **Insoluble Fiber** is mostly found in wholegrain cereals and products, and many vegetables. Its chief function is to keep bowel movements regular, so it helps to prevent problems like constipation, bowel cancer, and diverticular disease.

● **Soluble Fiber** is found in oats, legumes, fruits, and some vegetables. It forms a gummy substance in the gut and, if eaten regularly, can help to control blood sugar levels by slowing digestion and absorption of food, regulate appetite so we feel fuller longer, and reduce cholesterol levels – good news for people with diabetes. Foods rich in soluble fiber have a low GI (*see page 17*).

SOURCES OF FATS

The main sources of the four types of fat are:

Saturates
○ Fatty meats, lard, butter, cream, hard cheese, and whole milk
○ Pastries
○ Coconut oil and palm oil

Monounsaturates
○ Olive, rapeseed, and peanut oils
○ Avocados
○ Most nuts

Polyunsaturates
○ Omega 6: sunflower, corn, safflower, and soy oils and margarines; grapeseed oil; and sunflower and sesame seeds
○ Omega 3: oily fish; fish oils

Trans Fatty Acids
○ Hard margarines
○ Fast foods
○ Cookies, cakes, and pastries

BUYING & COOKING FOOD

THE VAST RANGE OF PROCESSED FOODS AVAILABLE TODAY CAN BE USED IN A HEALTHY, BALANCED DIET, PROVIDED THAT YOU HAVE SOME KNOW-HOW ABOUT READING THE LABELS. THE INGREDIENTS LABEL IS EASY TO UNDERSTAND, SINCE INGREDIENTS ARE ALWAYS LISTED IN ORDER OF WEIGHT, SO THAT THE MAIN INGREDIENT IS FIRST ON THE LIST. NUTRITIONAL LABELS ARE MORE COMPLICATED.

What the labels say When you read the nutrition information on food labels, you should consider how the food might fit into your overall diet. Some foods may look to be high in sugar, fat, or calories, but if they are eaten only in small amounts or occasionally, their fat, sugar, and calories can still fit into the overall balance of your diet. Foods that you eat regularly, or in larger amounts at any one time, affect the balance of your diet more. When buying them, it is worth looking for brands lower in fat, sugar, and salt. The nutrition information on food labels shows how much of a nutrient they will provide and allows you to compare the nutrient content of foods.

NUTRITION INFORMATION ON FOOD LABELS

These are the nutrients typically included on food labels, depending on their significance in the food being labeled. The "percent daily values" are based on a 2,000 calorie diet.

Energy (Kcals or Kj) The amount of energy, measured as calories that you will get from the food.

Fiber (g) This figure is the total amount of fiber in the food, including soluble and insoluble. Aim to eat around 24g of fiber each day.

Cholesterol (mg) The amount of cholesterol in the food per recommended serving size. Adults should not exceed 300mg daily.

Sodium (g) Most of the sodium in food comes from salt (sodium chloride). It is advisable to have no more than 2.4g sodium per day (equivalent to 6g salt).

Nutrition Facts

Serving size: 3 oz/84g	Amount per Serving	% Daily Value
Calories	140	
Total Fat	8g	12%
Saturated Fat	2.5g	12%
Polyunstaurated Fat	2.5g	
Monounsaturated Fat	3g	
Fiber		
Cholesterol	45mg	15%
Sodium	520mg	22%
Total Carbohydrate	2g	1%
Protein	14g	
Iron		6%

Protein (g) There is usually more than enough in the diet, so there is no need to pay too much attention to this (unless you are on a special, low-protein diet).

Iron 75mg of iron are suggested per day, but since various diets result in different iron absorptions, consult your doctor if you are anemic.

Fat (g) This figure is the total amount of fat in the food, and is sometimes broken down into saturates, monounsaturates, and polyunsaturates. Try to choose foods that are low in total fat and particularly in saturates. Choose oils and spreads that are rich in monounsaturates.

Total Carbohydrate (g) These are mainly starches and sugars (all types), given either as figures for each, or just as total carbohydrate. Try to choose foods that are higher in starchy carbohydrate than in sugars.

CHOOSING HEALTHIER ALTERNATIVES

When shopping for ready-made foods or for the ingredients for
your own cooking, always be on the lookout for healthier options –
that is, foods or ingredients that are lower in fat or sugar than the
traditional versions. You may find the following suggestions helpful.

HIGH-FAT FOODS	LOWER FAT OPTIONS
• Whole milk and dairy foods	• Low fat milks, yogurts, cottage cheese
• Hard cheeses	• Low fat Cheddar, Brie, or Edam cheeses; low-fat soft cheese
• Butter and margarine	• Low or reduced fat spreads low in saturates
• Fatty and processed meats	• Lean fresh meat (or meat trimmed of fat), ham, cold roast meat, lean back bacon
• Cheesy or oily sauces	• Vegetable-based sauces
• Salad dressings	• Fat-free, yogurt-based dressings; balsamic vinegar
• High-fat prepared meals	• Meals without pastry, cream or cheese sauces, with no more than 10–15g fat per serving
• Rich dairy desserts	• Light or low fat yogurts, mousses, rice pudding, custards, and cottage cheese (look for low-sugar types, too)
• Potato chips and salty snacks	• Homemade popcorn (no fat), homemade pita "chips", rice cakes, pretzels, bread sticks

HIGH-SUGAR FOODS	LOW-SUGAR OPTIONS
• Sugar, glucose, fructose	• Artificial (intense) sweetener
• Sodas, such as cola or tonic	• Diet, slimline, or one-cal sodas
• Soft drinks, cordials	• Sugar-free, low-calorie soft drinks or cordials
• Canned fruits	• Canned fruits in natural juice
• Sweet desserts	• Low- or reduced sugar or sugar-free rice puddings, whips, mousses, jellies, and custard
• Sweet cookies	• Plain or semi-sweet cookies
• Cakes	• Scones, fruit breads, fat-free puddings

MEAL PLANNING

FOOD CHOICE AND MEAL PLANNING ARE KEY
FACTORS IN MANAGING DIABETES. A BALANCED DIET
CAN HELP NOT ONLY LONG-TERM HEALTH–WEIGHT
MANAGEMENT AND CONTROL OF BLOOD LIPIDS
(FATS), BUT ALSO CONTROL OF GLUCOSE LEVELS
ON A DAY-TO-DAY BASIS.

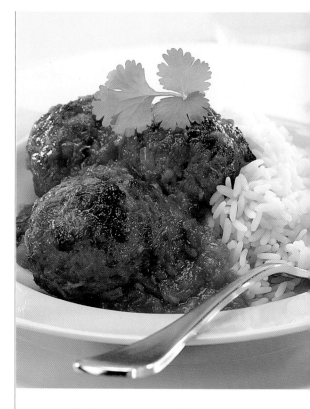

Regular meals

Eating regular meals based on starchy foods and serving starchy foods like bread, rice, potatoes, pasta, and cereals with meals is the best foundation for your diet. Start the day with breakfast, including cereal, fruits (fresh or dried), low-fat milk, toast, low fat spread, and preserves. Have a sandwich, filled roll or bagel, or some other snack to break up the day. Try to have a balanced main meal every day, avoiding fried dishes and pastry on a regular basis and eating plenty of starchy foods, vegetables, and fruits. To ensure that ready-made meals are balanced, serve them with starchy foods and extra vegetables or salads. End main meals with fruit-based desserts.

Balanced meals

A practical way to get a healthy balance to your eating is to think of a meal as a plate to be filled (see page 16). Fill half the plate with starchy food like bread, potatoes, pasta, or cereals. On the other half of the plate fill two-thirds with vegetables, salad, or fruits, and fill the remaining third with food that is a good source of protein, such as lean meat, fish, chicken, beans, tofu, or cheese. Include beans, wholewheat pasta, or brown rice in salads. Dairy products like cheese can be high in fat, so limit the amount you eat and use lower fat varieties if you are trying to reduce your overall calorie intake.

MIDWEEK DINNERS

These are good midweek meals for busy people. Quick and easy to prepare, they include dishes made in advance.

CHICKEN, LIMA BEAN,
TARRAGON & LEEK PIE (page 62)
served with vegetables or salad

SIMPLE CITRUS TERRINE (page 101)

PORK & CILANTRO MEATBALLS WITH
TOMATO SAUCE (page 66)
served with rice or pasta and salad

BLUEBERRY MERINGUE ICE CREAM
(page 92)

ABOVE *Pork & Cilantro Meatballs
with Tomato Sauce*

VEGETARIAN DINNERS

Although these satisfying two-course meals are planned for vegetarians, they will please the whole family.

CHARRED VEGETABLE PASTA *(page 72)*
served with bread and salad

BAKED PEACH PACKETS *(page 100)*

VEGETABLE CASSOULET *(page 70)*

APRICOT PUDDING *(page 105)*

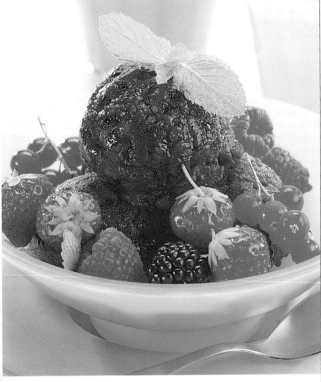

BELOW *Charred Vegetable Pasta*

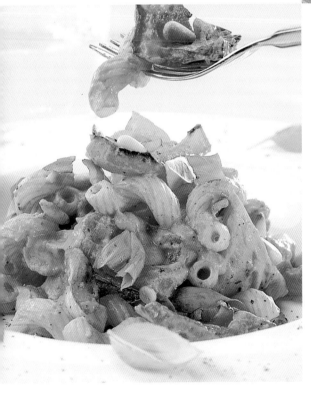

LOW-CALORIE MEALS

Meals such as these make cutting down on the calories to reduce your weight both easy and enjoyable.

STEAMED FISH PARCELS WITH HORSERADISH & TARTARE SAUCE *(page 64)* served with new potatoes and salad

SUMMER FRUIT SORBET *(page 90)*

SPINACH- & RICOTTA-FILLED CHICKEN *(page 57)* served with rice and vegetables

SPICED FRUIT KEBABS *(page 97)*

MARINATED TOFU STIR-FRY *(page 71)*

PAPAYA & PASSION FRUIT COMPOTE WITH BASIL *(page 101)*

ABOVE *Summer Fruit Sorbet*

The serving suggestions included in the menus on these pages will help you to plan balanced meals. If you have dishes with a high fat content, combine them with plenty of vegetables and low fat, starchy foods. Plan meals so that the different dishes and courses complement each other nutritionally.

Snacks

If you are taking insulin you may need to use snacks as a means of spreading your carbohydrate intake out evenly in order to help keep your glucose levels within a reasonable range. Fresh fruits are an ideal carbohydrate boost – and they are fat-free.

Planning meals

A dietitian will help you to adjust eating habits and food choice and will give guidance on specific dietary goals. Use the menus here to help you to understand more about balancing choices.

Adapting recipes

Favorite recipes need not be abandoned because you need to follow a diabetes diet. There are two main ways in which you can adapt recipes and use them in menus similar to those here:

● **Cut down on fat** Opt for low fat or fat-free ways of cooking, such as microwaving, baking, broiling, poaching, and steaming; stir-fry in non-stick pans; roast on a rack. Use low fat dairy products in place of whole milk, cream, cheeses, and yogurts. Remove skin, the fattest part, from poultry. Choose lean cuts of red meat and trim off as much fat as possible.

● **Reduce the sugar content of recipes** Use dried fruits in place of some or all of the sugar in foods like cheesecakes, non-baked goods, and heavy-textured baked goods such as fruit breads. Reduce the sugar content by half in baking: while some sugar is needed for good rising and correct texture, half the recipe quantity will still give good results. Use artificial sweeteners in sprinkle, liquid, or tablet form to sweeten foods after cooking.

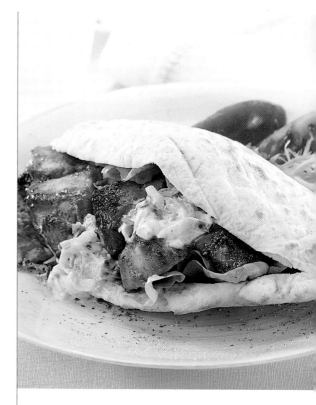

LIGHT LUNCHES

Midday meals need not be big to be satisfying, as the suggestions here demonstrate.

PITA POCKETS STUFFED WITH CHICKEN TIKKA & RAITA (*page 48*)
with a piece of fruit

STEAK SANDWICH (*page 52*)

BRUNCHES

POACHED EGGS & PROSCIUTTO ON ENGLISH MUFFINS (*page 45*)

BLT BAGEL WITH HERB CREME FRAICHE (*page 53*)

ABOVE Pita Pockets Stuffed with Chicken Tikka & Raita

DINNER PARTIES

These splendid three-course meals will
impress all lovers of good food.

ZUCCHINI & PEA SOUP WITH
MINT PESTO *(page 33)*

PORK STUFFED WITH BLUE CHEESE & SAGE
(page 67) served with PUREED CELERIAC
(page 89) and vegetables

FRUIT SABAYON *(page 104)*

SMOKED SALMON & TARRAGON PATE *(page 34)*

PAN-FRIED DUCK BREASTS WITH MANGO
SALSA *(page 54)* served with SAUTEED
CABBAGE WITH SEEDS *(page 84)* and new potatoes

SPICED POACHED PEARS WITH VANILLA
MINT CREAM *(page 102)*

BELOW *Spiced Poached Pears with Vanilla Mint Cream*

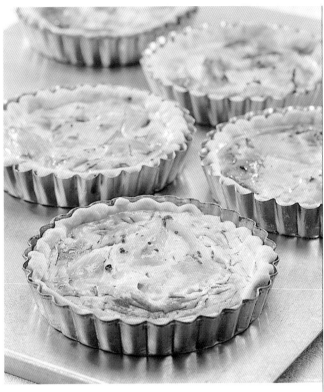

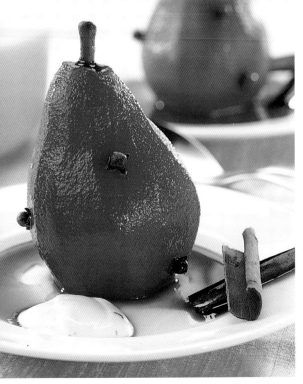

BUFFET

This is a splendid buffet spread, chosen
from all sections of this book.

HOT CHILI SHRIMP *(page 36)*

CHICKEN & BEEF SATAY WITH PEANUT
DIPPING SAUCE *(page 38)*

SUPER-SIMPLE SMOKED SALMON
TARTLETS *(page 46)*

SPINACH TORTILLA *(page 49)*

POTATO WEDGES *(page 45)*

LAMB & FLAGEOLET BEAN SALAD *(page 53)*

MEDITERRANEAN BREAD SALAD *(page 83)*

PESTO VEGETABLE KEBABS *(page 83)*

BAKED ST. CLEMENT'S CHEESECAKE *(page 106)*

ABOVE *Super-simple Smoked Salmon Tartlets*

OUT & ABOUT

EATING AT REGULAR TIMES IS VERY IMPORTANT. THIS MEANS THAT IF YOU ARE EATING AWAY

FROM HOME, WHETHER FOR JUST AN EVENING OR DURING THE COURSE OF A LONGER

VACATION, YOU WILL NEED TO THINK ABOUT THE MEALS YOU WILL BE EATING AND

DO SOME PLANNING AHEAD.

MENU DECODER

Use this guide to eating-place menu descriptions to sort out the lower fat dishes on the menu from those higher in fat.

Lower fat dishes
- Steamed
- Poached
- Broiled
- Flame-broiled
- Char-broiled
- Baked
- Cooked in its own juice
- Pomodoro (tomato sauce)
- Wine sauce
- Stir-fried

Higher fat dishes
- Deep-fried
- En croute
- Hollandaise
- Creamy
- Au gratin
- Crispy
- Coconut cream/milk
- Sautéed
- Béchamel
- Pan-fried

Away from home

If you are going to eat later than you usually do, you will probably need to have a snack at your usual mealtime to prevent a hypoglycemic episode (*see page 13*). Always carry a carbohydrate-rich snack with you when away from home and have something to hand when traveling. This is in case your usual meal or snack time is delayed, or you are unexpectedly more active (you need to eat some form of carbohydrate before any exercise since it lowers glucose levels). If you are meeting friends for a drink, it is important not to miss meals or snacks because alcohol can lower glucose levels and increase the risk of a hypoglycemic episode. If your diabetes is treated by diet alone or by diet and tablets, the exact time you eat is not so crucial and a one- or two-hour delay in meal times should not upset your diabetes control. Your diabetes care team can give you good advice about managing your diabetes away from home.

Eating out

These days, people may eat out several times a week, whether it is having a meal at work, a quick sandwich with a friend, or dinner after a trip to the movies. For a person with diabetes, making wise choices when eating away from home does make a difference. Here is how everything can be kept in balance:

- **Ask for extra bread** but decline butter – enjoy all kinds of breads, from wholewheat varieties to those served with Asian meals.

- **Ask for a pitcher of water** to quench your thirst.

- **Order a maximum of two courses** and ensure that at least one of them is based on vegetables, seafood, or fruits.

- **Beware portion sizes,** which are often much bigger or have too little carbohydrate compared with what you would serve yourself at home.

- **Avoid deep-fried and battered dishes** or meals smothered in cheese or cream sauce (*see Menu Decoder, left, for more low fat dishes*). Ask for sauces to be served in separate dishes so that you can control the amounts of sauce that are put on your food.

● **Exert your customer rights,** requesting changes to how dishes are prepared, if necessary: grilled or poached fish rather than fried; no added fat to vegetables or broiled or steamed foods; new or baked potatoes rather than roast, fried, or sautéed; steamed rice rather than fried; larger portions of vegetables, salads, potatoes, rice, or pasta; no cream in sauces; no butter or mayonnaise; oil-free salad dressings.

● **Aim for healthy proportions** and choose a good basis of rice, pasta, bread, potatoes, or noodles; modest amounts of protein (meat, chicken, fish, eggs, beans), and plenty of vegetables or salad.

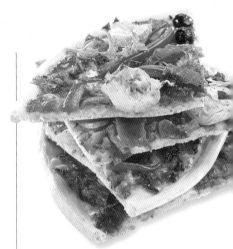

GOOD PIZZA CHOICE
Careful choice of toppings can give you an away-from-home pizza similar to the Fantastic Four Seasons Pizza (recipe, page 50).

Better fast food choices

● **Burger restaurants** Plain hamburgers or cheeseburgers; flame-broiled chicken burgers; no mayonnaise; orange juice; diet drinks.

● **Fish and chips** Thick chips (they have less fat than fries); puréed peas (for fiber). Remove some batter from the fish.

● **Sandwiches, rolls, and bagels** Omit butter or mayonnaise; good fillings are salad, plus tuna, salmon, roasted lean meat, ham, chicken, turkey, egg, Edam, Brie, low fat cream cheese, or hummus.

● **Pizza** With vegetables, ham, tuna, or seafood toppings rather than pepperoni or extra cheese. Choose fat-free dressings from the salad bar.

● **Snacks** Fresh fruits or fruit salads; yogurts or rice puddings; cereal bars; blueberry muffins; fruit scones; large pretzels.

A HEALTHY BAGEL
Duplicate the filling in the BLT Bagel with Herb Crème Fraîche (recipe, page 53) when choosing fast food away from home.

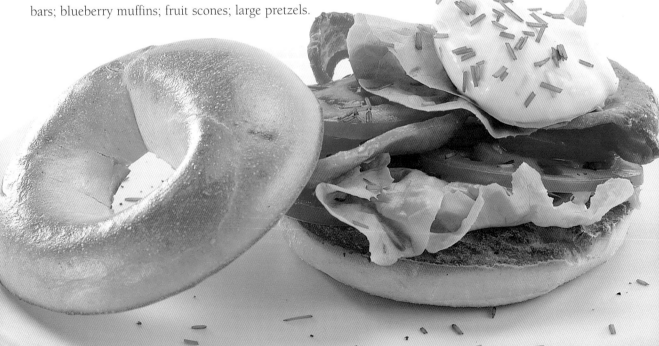

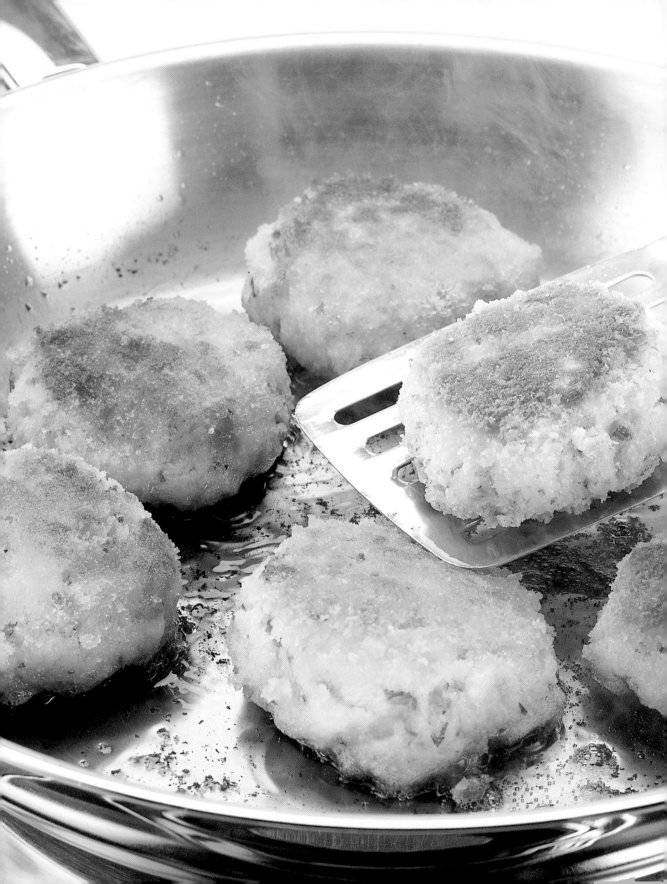

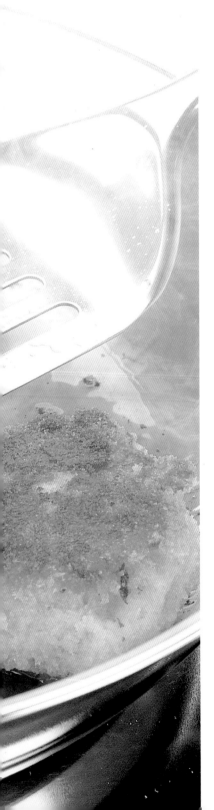

RECIPES

WITH OVER 100 ENTICING RECIPES, THIS SECTION GUARANTEES MAKING A *diet plan* FOR DIABETES SATISFYINGLY SIMPLE. EACH RECIPE INCLUDES A *nutritional analysis* TO HELP YOU SET UP A HEALTHY, BALANCED DIET, AND THERE ARE MANY TIPS ON SERVING, PREPARATION, AND *key healthy foods*. APPEALING TO THE WHOLE FAMILY, WHETHER DEALING WITH DIABETES OR NOT, THE RECIPES ARE A FINE SOURCE OF *delicious* FOOD FOR ALL OCCASIONS.

LEFT: SPICY CRAB CAKES *(see page 42)*

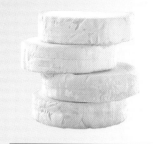

GOAT CHEESE CROSTINI WITH HAZELNUT SALSA

6 thick slices French bread
2 x 3¹/₂oz (100g) goat cheeses,
each cut into 3 slices
2oz (60g) mixed salad greens
orange peel, to garnish (optional)

FOR THE SALSA
1¹/₄ cups (30g) hazelnuts, toasted
4 tbsp fresh parsley
1 garlic clove
grated peel and juice of 1 orange
1 tbsp balsamic vinegar

★ STAR INGREDIENT
Goat and cow's milks have similar nutritional compositions, but because of the higher water content of goat cheese, it contains less fat than cheese made from cow's milk, like Cheddar.

EACH SERVING PROVIDES:
- ○ Calories 150
- ○ Protein 7g
- ○ Carbohydrate 14g
  Fiber 1g
- ○ Total Fat 8g
  Saturated Fat 3g
- ○ Sodium 256mg

SERVING TIP
Prepare the salsa in advance and keep it chilled in the refrigerator until needed.

Preparation Time: 15 minutes
Serves: 6

① First, make the salsa. Put the nuts in a blender or food processor, add the remaining ingredients, and blend for about 15 seconds. Transfer the salsa to a small saucepan and heat it through gently.

② Meanwhile, toast each bread slice on one side. Place a slice of goat cheese on the untoasted side of each piece of bread. Put all 6 slices under a preheated hot broiler and broil for 1–2 minutes, until the cheese is golden and bubbling.

③ Divide the salad greens among 6 plates and top with a cheese toast, garnished, if liked, with strips of orange peel. Serve with the warm salsa, either spooned over the crostini or served separately.

APPETIZERS

Vegetables make a good foundation for many starters and soups. Serve them raw as crudités and salads, or cooked in soups, terrines, and dips. If an appetizer includes only a few carbohydrates, serve it with plenty of bread.

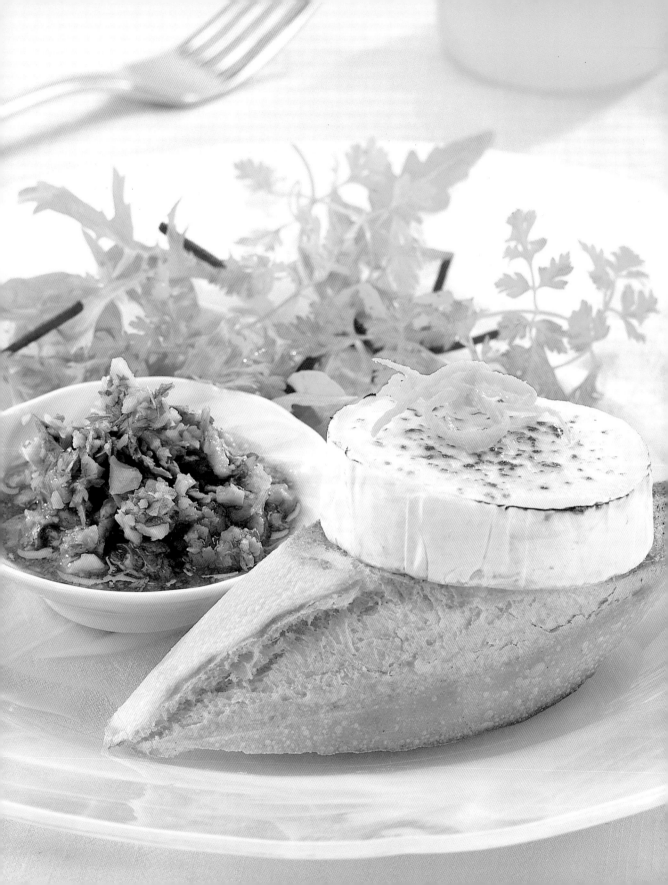

APRICOTS & PROSCIUTTO WITH GINGER DRESSING

EACH SERVING PROVIDES:

○ Calories 65

○ Protein 5g

○ Carbohydrate 3g
  Fiber 1g

○ Total Fat 3g
  Saturated Fat 1g

○ Sodium 305mg

SERVING TIP
Serve this with an Italian bread, such as Ciabatta or sun-dried tomato bread.

Preparation Time: 10 minutes
Serves: 6

¹/₂ bunch (60g) watercress
6 large fresh apricots, halved and stoned
3oz (90g) prosciutto, sliced

FOR THE DRESSING
1 piece preserved ginger, chopped
1 tbsp syrup from the ginger jar
1 tbsp balsamic vinegar
1 tbsp olive oil
salt and freshly ground black pepper

Divide the watercress among 6 serving plates. Put 2 apricot halves on top of the watercress on each plate, then cover with the prosciutto ham. Whisk together the ingredients for the dressing and drizzle over the apricots and prosciutto.

VARIATION
Classic Italian Starter Use a canteloupe, peeled, seeded, and cut into 6 wedges, in place of the apricots.

CRISPY BACON, AVOCADO & ARUGULA SALAD

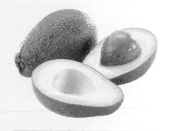

✳ STAR INGREDIENT
Avocado, unlike other fruits, contains some fat; it is monounsaturated fat, however, which is better for the heart than saturated fats.

EACH SERVING PROVIDES:

○ Calories 156

○ Protein 8g

○ Carbohydrate 2g
  Fiber 2g

○ Total Fat 12g
  Saturated Fat 3g

○ Sodium 545mg

Preparation Time: 15 minutes'
Serves: 4

4 strips lean back bacon
1 avocado, peeled and sliced
1 bunch (60g) arugula
100g (3¹/₂oz) cherry tomatoes, halved

FOR THE DRESSING
2 sun-dried tomatoes in oil, drained and chopped
2 tbsp oil from the sun-dried tomatoes
1 tbsp balsamic vinegar
1 tsp sugar

1 Broil the bacon strips under a preheated broiler until crisp. Drain the bacon on paper towels, then roughly chop it.

2 Put the bacon, avocado, arugula, and cherry tomatoes in a serving bowl and toss together gently.

3 Whisk together the ingredients for the dressing, drizzle over the salad, and serve.

WHITE BEAN SOUP

EACH SERVING PROVIDES:

○ Calories 150

○ Protein 8g

○ Carbohydrate 20g
Fiber 7g

○ Total Fat 4g
Saturated Fat 1g

○ Sodium 567mg

PREPARATION TIP
Reconstituted dried butter beans may be used for this soup. Soak 1lb (500g) dried beans overnight, drain, and cook in fresh water for about 1 hour, until tender.

Preparation Time: 30 minutes
Serves: 4

2¹/₂lb (1.25kg) canned white beans, rinsed and drained

3³/₄ cups (900ml) vegetable stock

2 tbsp olive oil

3 garlic cloves, finely sliced

6 tomatoes, finely chopped

2 tbsp chopped fresh sage

salt and freshly ground black pepper, to taste

1 Put the beans and stock in a medium saucepan, bring to a boil, reduce the heat, cover, and simmer for 10 minutes.

2 Use a slotted spoon to take about a third of the beans from the saucepan and set aside. Transfer the remaining beans and the cooking liquid to a food processor or blender and process into a smooth purée. Return the bean purée and the whole beans to the pan.

3 Heat the oil in a saucepan; add the garlic, and fry gently until golden. Add the tomatoes and sage, cover the pan, and simmer for 5 minutes.

4 Stir the tomato mixture into the bean mixture and heat through. Season to taste before serving.

ZUCCHINI & PEA SOUP WITH MINT PESTO

EACH SERVING PROVIDES:

○ Calories 200

○ Protein 7g

○ Carbohydrate 10g
Fiber 5g

○ Total Fat 12g
Saturated Fat 2g

○ Sodium 6mg

NUTRITION TIP
Soups based on vegetables, such as this one, are generally high in fibre and low in fat.

Preparation Time: 20 minutes
Serves: 4

1 tsp olive oil

1 onion, chopped

1 garlic clove, crushed

2 large zucchini, grated

2 cups (250g) peas, defrosted if frozen

2¹/₂ cups (600ml) vegetable stock

salt and freshly ground black pepper

FOR THE PESTO

8 tbsp chopped fresh mint

1 garlic clove

3 tbsp walnuts, toasted

2 tbsp olive oil

salt and freshly ground black pepper, to taste

1 Heat the oil in a large saucepan. Add the onion, garlic, and zucchini, and fry gently for 3–4 minutes, until beginning to soften.

2 Add the peas and stock to the pan, bring to a boil, reduce the heat, and simmer for 5 minutes. Season well.

3 Put the ingredients for the pesto in a blender and process until combined, but still retaining a slightly rough texture.

4 Serve the soup hot or chilled, with a spoonful of mint pesto on top.

EACH SERVING PROVIDES:

○ Calories 137

○ Protein 6g

○ Carbohydrate 22g
  Fiber 3g

○ Total Fat 3g
  Saturated Fat 0g

○ Sodium 165mg

SERVING TIP
This soup freezes well. Use it
within 3 months of freezing.

**Preparation Time: 45–50
minutes
Serves: 6**

SPICY LENTIL SOUP

1 tbsp olive oil
2 garlic cloves, crushed
1 large onion, chopped
1 inch (2.5cm) piece fresh ginger,
peeled and grated
1 parsnip, chopped
1 large potato, chopped
2 sticks celery, chopped

2 tbsp medium curry paste
1/2 cup (100g) red lentils
6 1/4 cups (1.5 liters) vegetable stock
1 1/2 cups (400g) canned coconut milk
grated peel and juice of 1/2 lemon
1/2 cup (15g) chopped cilantro
salt and freshly ground
black pepper, to taste

1 Heat the oil in a large saucepan. Add the garlic, onion, and ginger,
and fry gently for 2–3 minutes.

2 Add the parsnip, potato, and celery to the pan and continue to fry
gently for 3 minutes. Stir the curry paste through the vegetables and
cook for a further minute.

3 Add the lentils and stock to the pan. Bring to a boil, reduce the
heat, cover, and simmer for 25 minutes, or until the lentils are tender.

4 Pour the mixture into a blender or food processor, and process until
smooth. Return it to the pan, add the remaining ingredients, with
seasoning to taste, and heat through before serving.

EACH SERVING PROVIDES:

○ Calories 73

○ Protein 6g

○ Carbohydrate 0g
  Fiber 0g

○ Total Fat 5g
  Saturated Fat 3g

○ Sodium 395mg

NUTRITION TIP
Reduce the fat and calorie
contents of dishes by using
low-fat dairy products, as here.

**Preparation Time: 5 minutes
Serves: 8**

SMOKED SALMON & TARRAGON PATE

1 cup (200g) low fat cream cheese
grated peel and juice of 1 lemon
5oz (150g) smoked salmon
2 tbsps chopped fresh tarragon
2 tbsp low fat crème fraîche
salt and freshly ground black pepper, to taste

1 Put all the ingredients for the pâté in a blender or food processor
and process until almost smooth.

2 Put the pâté in a bowl, cover, and chill until required.

CHICKEN LIVER PATE

1lb (500g) chicken livers
2 tbsp (30g) butter
1 onion, cut into wedges
3 garlic cloves

4 tbsp low fat crème fraîche
1 tbsp brandy
salt and freshly ground black pepper, to taste

1 Preheat the oven to 400°F/200°C. Put the chicken livers, butter, onion, and garlic in an ovenproof dish. Roast in the preheated oven for 25–30 minutes, until the onion is cooked.

2 Transfer the mixture to a food processor or blender, add the remaining ingredients, and process until smooth.

3 Taste the pâté and add seasoning, if necessary. Transfer to a pâté dish or bowl, cover, and chill in the refrigerator until required.

EGGPLANT PATE

GOOD EITHER AS A VEGETARIAN STARTER OR AS A DIP WITH DRINKS,

THIS PATE MAY BE EATEN EITHER WARM OR COLD. SERVE IT WITH

TOASTED PITA BREAD OR BREADSTICKS.

3 large eggplants, pricked all over
1 tbsp olive oil
1 red chili, finely chopped
1 tbsp black mustard seeds
*1 inch (2.5cm) piece fresh ginger,
peeled and grated*
2 tbsp creamed coconut
4 tbsp chopped cilantro

1 Preheat the oven to 400°F/200°C. Lay the eggplants on a baking sheet and bake for 40–45 minutes, until tender. Cool, then halve them lengthways. Scoop out the flesh and discard the skin.

2 Heat the oil in a heavy-based saucepan, add the chili, mustard seeds, and ginger, and fry gently for 1 minute.

3 Stir in the eggplant flesh and the remaining ingredients, breaking up the eggplant flesh, and heat the pâté through. Serve the pâté warm, or let it cool before serving.

EACH SERVING PROVIDES:

○ Calories 97

○ Protein 10g

○ Carbohydrate 2g
Fiber 0g

○ Total Fat 5g
Saturated Fat 3g

○ Sodium 69mg

Preparation Time: 35–40 minutes
Serves: 8

✳ **STAR INGREDIENT**
Creamed coconut is high in saturated fat, but is acceptable in this recipe since only a small amount is used.

EACH SERVING PROVIDES:

○ Calories 74

○ Protein 2g

○ Carbohydrate 4g
Fiber 3g

○ Total Fat 6g
Saturated Fat 3g

○ Sodium 3mg

Preparation Time: 55–60 minutes
Serves: 4

SERVING TIP
These spicy shrimp are also delicious served cold (tail shells removed) on cocktail sticks with cubes of melon.

Preparation Time: 5 minutes,
plus 1 hour marinating
Serves: 4

Illustrated right

HOT CHILI SHRIMP

2 garlic cloves, crushed
grated peel and juice of 1 lime
1 large red chili, finely chopped
13oz (400g) large shrimp,
shelled, with tails left intact
1 tbsp light vegetable oil
1 tbsp honey
3 tbsp chopped cilantro

1 Put the garlic, lime peel and juice, and chili in a bowl and mix well together. Stir in the shrimp and let them marinate for about 1 hour.

2 Heat the oil in a frying pan or wok. Lift the shrimp from the marinade with a slotted spoon and put carefully into the pan. Cook gently for 1–2 minutes, turning in the pan, until hot.

3 Pour any remaining marinade into the pan, with the honey and cilantro, and heat through. Turn the shrimp into a warmed serving bowl or on to individual plates and serve immediately.

NUTRITION TIP
Pastry is high in fat, so make pies and tarts with a single, rather than double, crust.

Preparation Time: 30 minutes
Makes: 20

BRIE & TOMATO TARTLETS

8oz (250g) puff pastry, thawed if frozen
3 tbsp pesto
4 tomatoes, sliced
4oz (125g) brie, sliced
salt and freshly ground black pepper,
to taste
fresh basil, to garnish

1 Preheat the oven to 400°F/200°C. Roll out the pastry on a lightly floured surface to a rectangle about 9 x 11in (23 x 28cm). Cut into 20 rounds with a 2in (5cm) pastry cutter.

2 Put a small amount of pesto on each pastry round, then top with a slice of tomato and a slice of brie. Season well.

3 Place the pastry rounds on a baking sheet and bake for about 15 minutes, or until golden. Serve garnished with the basil.

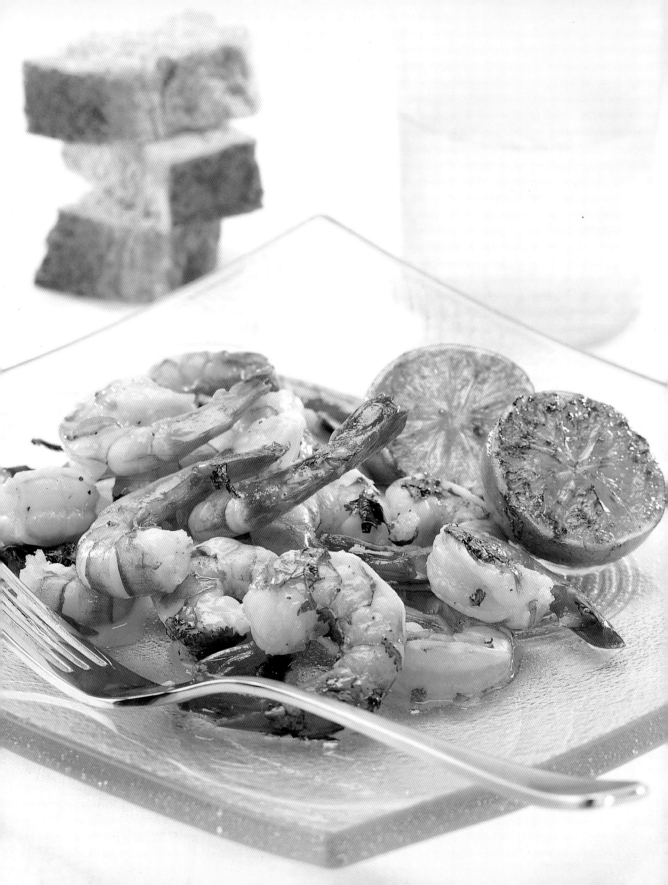

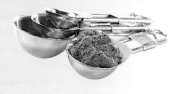

EACH SERVING PROVIDES:

○ Calories 207

○ Protein 20g

○ Carbohydrate 4g
   Fiber 1g

○ Total Fat 12g
   Saturated Fat 3g

○ Sodium 710mg

SERVING TIP
This peanut sauce also makes
a good accompaniment for
vegetarian dishes such as
vegetable kebabs.

Preparation Time: 15–20
minutes, plus 30 minutes
marinating
Serves: 6

CHICKEN & BEEF SATAY WITH PEANUT DIPPING SAUCE

IN THIS RECIPE, SUCCULENT, BITE-SIZED PIECES OF MEAT ARE
ACCOMPANIED BY A MILDLY SPICY PEANUT SAUCE. THIS MAKES AN
EXCELLENT DISH FOR SERVING AT COCKTAIL PARTIES OR BUFFET MEALS.

*7oz (200g) boneless, skinless chicken breast
halves, cut into strips
7oz (200g) sirloin steak, cut into strips
2 garlic cloves, crushed
4 tbsp soy sauce*

*FOR THE PEANUT SAUCE
1 tsp olive oil
¹/₂ onion, finely chopped
1 tbsp medium-strength curry paste
1 tsp chili powder
6 tbsp crunchy peanut butter
²/₃ cup (150ml) low fat milk*

1 Thread the chicken and beef pieces on to small wooden skewers
or cocktail sticks. Place in a non-metallic dish.

2 Mix together the garlic and soy sauce, pour over the meat, and
leave to marinate for 30 minutes.

3 For the peanut sauce, heat the oil in a non-stick frying pan, fry
the onion for 2 minutes, add the curry paste and chili powder, and
continue to fry gently for 1 minute. Add the peanut butter and milk
and heat through. Transfer the sauce to a serving dish.

4 Put the skewers of meat under a preheated broiler and cook for
4–5 minutes, turning occasionally until cooked. Transfer the skewers
to a serving platter and serve with the peanut sauce.

ANTIPASTI

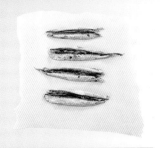

A SELECTION OF ANTIPASTI FOODS, LIKE THOSE SUGGESTED HERE,

MAKES AN EASY-TO-MAKE AND VERY EFFECTIVE APPETIZER, FROM

WHICH GUESTS CAN HELP THEMSELVES.

Suggested Ingredients
marinated peppers
artichoke hearts
marinated olives
selection of cold sliced meats
selection of pickles
selection of tomatoes
fresh broiled anchovies
canned white beans or other legumes

✴ STAR INGREDIENT
Fresh anchovies are lower in fat and contain less salt than canned ones.

PREPARATION TIP
For an antipasti first course that requires little time spent on it on the day, choose ingredients that can be prepared the day before or that require little attention apart from setting out on a plate and garnishing with fresh herbs.

SERVING TIP
Although some of the foods suggested here may be high in fat, guests can select what they want and balance their choices. When planning an antipasti course, allow 3 or 4 items per person.

• **Marinated peppers** Halve 2 or 3 peppers, core and seed them (*see page 71*), and broil them until the skins are charred. Put the peppers in a plastic bag for 3 or 4 minutes, then peel off the skins and slice the flesh. Drizzle with a little oil and sprinkle with chopped garlic and fresh herbs.

• **Artichoke hearts** Use ready-made artichoke hearts, widely available canned or in jars of oil, garnished with fresh herbs.

• **Olives** Marinating gives olives extra flavor and succulence. Put them in a screw-top or preserving jar with a little olive oil or a lighter vegetable oil, fresh herbs, 1 or 2 garlic cloves, and a red chili. Leave for 2–3 days, occasionally shaking the jar gently.

• **Sliced meats and pickles** Include ham or salami among the meats, and gherkins and small onions among the pickles selection.

• **Tomatoes** Include both sun-dried and fresh cherry tomatoes.

• **Legumes** Drain and rinse a can of your chosen beans, stir through a little Fat-free Dressing (*see below*), and season well.

Fat-free Dressing Mix together ⅔ cup (150ml) apple juice, 2 tablespoons white wine vinegar, 1 tablespoon honey, and 1 tablespoon wholegrain mustard.

TEN-MINUTE CHINESE CHICKEN NOODLES

STIR-FRYING IS A QUICK AND HEALTHY METHOD OF COOKING. ONLY A SMALL AMOUNT OF OIL IS USED, AND THE SHORT COOKING TIME ENSURES THAT THE VITAMIN CONTENT OF FOOD IS NOT DEPLETED.

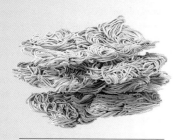

✱ STAR INGREDIENT
Egg noodles make perfect pasta dishes when a quick meal is needed.

EACH SERVING PROVIDES:

○ Calories 438

○ Protein 30g

○ Carbohydrate 63g
  Fiber 3g

○ Total Fat 9g
  Saturated Fat 2g

○ Sodium 947mg

SERVING TIP
Serve this dish with bread and a green, leafy salad for a quick, substantial meal.

Preparation Time: 20 minutes
Serves: 3

1 tsp sesame oil
1 boneless, skinless chicken breast half,
about 4oz (125g), finely sliced
1 bunch scallions, sliced
100g (3½oz) snow peas, trimmed and halved
1 red chili, finely chopped
2 tbsp dark soy sauce
2½oz (75g) cooked ham, chopped
2 cups (250g) egg noodles
2 tbsp chopped cilantro

1 Heat the oil in a non-stick frying pan or wok, add the chicken pieces, and stir-fry for 2–3 minutes.

2 Add the scallions, snow peas, and chilli, and continue to stir-fry for 2 minutes. Stir in the soy sauce and ham.

3 Meanwhile, cook the noodles. Drop them into a large saucepan of boiling water, reduce the heat, and simmer for 3–4 minutes. Drain well.

4 Toss together the noodles, chicken mixture, and cilantro, turn into a warmed serving bowl, and serve immediately.

SNACKS

However quick and easy they may be to prepare, light meals and snacks should still incorporate starchy staples like bread, rice, pasta, and potatoes. There is a varied selection of all these foods in the wonderfully flavorsome recipes in this chapter.

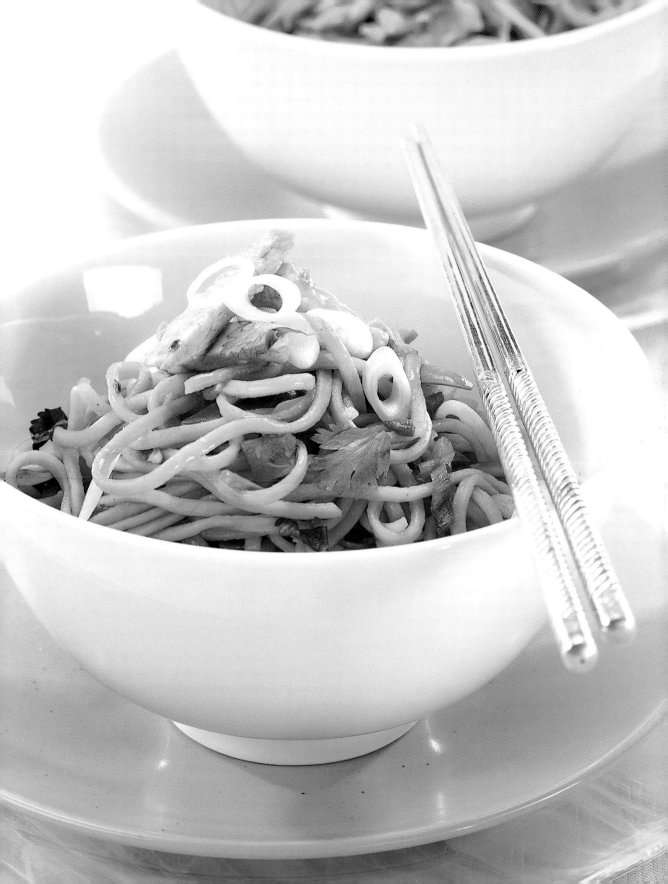

SMOKED MACKEREL PASTA

3 cups (375g) dried pasta
1 tsp oil
1 onion, sliced
4 cups (275g) mixed mushrooms, sliced
2 peppered smoked mackerel fillets,
each about 3oz (90g), skinned and flaked
6 tbsp low fat crème fraîche
2 tbsp chopped fresh herbs
salt and freshly ground black pepper,
to taste

1 Slide the pasta into a large pan of boiling water and cook for 8–10 minutes,.or until just tender.

2 Meanwhile, heat the oil in a non-stick frying pan, add the onion and fry gently for 2–3 minutes, or until softened. Add the mushrooms and continue to fry gently for a further 3 minutes.

3 Drain the pasta and return it to the pan. Stir in the onion mixture, mackerel, crème fraîche, and herbs. Season well, heat through gently, and turn into a warmed serving bowl. Serve at once.

Sidebar (Smoked Mackerel Pasta)

EACH SERVING PROVIDES:

○ Calories 385

○ Protein 15g

○ Carbohydrate 50g
Fiber 3g

○ Total Fat 15g
Saturated Fat 4g

○ Sodium 266mg

NUTRITION TIP
Pasta is an ideal starchy food to use as a basis for meals, because it has a low glycemic index (*see page 17*), which helps to keep blood glucose levels steady.

Preparation Time: 25 minutes
Serves: 6

SPICY CRAB CAKES

12oz (375g) fresh crabmeat or
same quantity canned crabmeat
3 cups (250g) potatoes, peeled,
cooked,and mashed
1 tbsp Thai green curry paste
3 tbsp chopped cilantro

1 bunch scallions, finely sliced
grated peel and juice of ½ lemon
flour, for coating
2 eggs, beaten
1½ cups (150g) fresh breadcrumbs
3 tbsp oil

1 In a large bowl, mix together the crab, mashed potatoes, curry paste, cilantro, scallions, and lemon peel and juice.

2 Form the mixture into 18 cakes, each about ½in (1cm) thick. Coat the cakes in the flour, then in the egg, then in the breadcrumbs.

3 Heat the oil in a non-stick frying pan and fry the crab cakes on medium heat in batches until golden, turning them once or twice in the oil. Drain on paper towels and serve while still hot.

Sidebar (Spicy Crab Cakes)

EACH SERVING PROVIDES:

○ Calories 181

○ Protein 17g

○ Carbohydrate 24g
Fiber 1g

○ Total Fat 3g
Saturated Fat 1g

○ Sodium 473mg

PREPARATION TIP
Canned fish or shellfish meat has the same nutritional value as fresh seafood, but look out for added salt or oil.

Preparation Time: 25–30 minutes
Serves: 6

Illustrated on pages 28–29

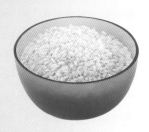

TOMATO & HERB RISOTTO

STARCHY FOODS LIKE RICE MAKE AN EXCELLENT BASIS FOR MEALS.

SERVE THIS RISOTTO WITH A GREEN, LEAFY SALAD.

1 tsp olive oil
1 small onion, finely chopped
2 garlic cloves, crushed
1³/₄ cups (375g) risotto rice
²/₃ cup (150ml) dry white wine
5 cups (1.2 liters) boiling vegetable stock
1 cup (275g) cherry tomatoes, halved
4 sun-dried tomatoes, chopped
3 tbsp tomato purée
3 tbsp grated fresh Parmesan
*4 tbsp chopped fresh herbs,
such as parsley, rosemary, and basil*
salt and freshly ground black pepper, to taste

1 Heat the oil in a large, non-stick frying pan. Add the onion and garlic and stir-fry gently for 2 minutes. Stir in the rice, turning it to coat in the oil. Add the wine, bring to the boil, reduce the heat, and simmer until the rice has absorbed the liquid.

2 Add a ladle of boiling stock and simmer until absorbed, stirring continuously. Continue this process until all the stock has been used, adding the tomatoes and tomato purée with the last ladle of stock.

3 Stir the Parmesan and herbs through the rice, taste and adjust the seasoning, if necessary, and serve.

VARIATIONS

Mushroom Risotto Fry 6 cups (500g) mixed fresh mushrooms gently in 1 tablespoon olive oil until tender and add to the pan in place of the tomatoes and tomato purée.

Vegetable Risotto Add 4 cups (300g) mixed spring vegetables, such as peas, asparagus, and green beans, trimmed and blanched, if necessary, in place of the tomatoes and tomato purée. Add them with the final ladle of stock.

✳ STAR INGREDIENT
All varieties of rice have a similar nutritional composition, although brown rice is higher in fiber than other varieties.

EACH SERVING PROVIDES:

○ Calories 179

○ Protein 6g

○ Carbohydrate 20g
   Fiber 1g

○ Total Fat 7g
   Saturated Fat 2g

○ Sodium 181mg

NUTRITION TIP
Parmesan is a high-fat cheese but, as it has a strong flavor and can be grated finely, only small amounts are needed.

Preparation Time: 35–40 minutes
Serves: 4

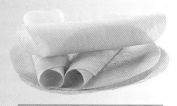

✻ STAR INGREDIENT
Spring roll wrappers are sold in supermarkets and Chinese food stores. Use filo pastry if they are unavailable.

EACH SERVING PROVIDES:

○ Calories 60

○ Protein 5g

○ Carbohydrate 5g
  Fiber 0g

○ Total Fat 2g
  Saturated Fat 0g

○ Sodium 17mg

NUTRITION TIP
Blood glucose levels (*see page 10*) are not harmed when foods with a high sugar content, like honey, are used in savory sauces.

Preparation Time: 45 minutes
Makes: 20

Spring Rolls with Chili & Cilantro Dipping Sauce

SPRING ROLLS ARE GENERALLY HIGH IN FAT SINCE THEY ARE DEEP-FRIED. IN THIS RECIPE, THE WRAPPERS ARE LIGHTLY BRUSHED WITH OIL, THEN BAKED TO MAKE THEM LOWER IN FAT.

1 cup (300g) egg noodles
3 tbsp olive oil
2 garlic cloves, crushed
2 boneless, skinless chicken breast halves,
each about 4oz (125g), cut into thin strips
6–8 scallions, finely sliced
1 large carrot, grated
1 cup (125g) beansprouts
1 tsp dried chili flakes
20 spring roll wrappers
2 eggs, beaten

For the Dip
2 tbsp honey
2 tbsp chili sauce
2 tbsp chopped cilantro

1 Cook the noodles in a large saucepan of boiling water for 3–4 minutes. Drain them well, then cut into 2in (5cm) lengths.

2 Heat 1 teaspoon of the oil in a frying pan. Add the garlic and fry gently for 1 minute. Add the chicken strips and continue to fry for 3 minutes, until cooked. Stir in the scallions, carrot, beansprouts, and chili flakes and continue to cook for 1 minute.

3 Preheat the oven to 400°F/200°C. Brush the spring roll wrappers on one side with a little beaten egg. Spoon a little filling on to each wrapper and roll up, making sure that the filling is completely enclosed. Brush each spring roll with a little oil and place on a baking sheet. Bake for 10–12 minutes, or until golden.

4 In a small bowl, mix together all the ingredients for the chili dip. Serve it with the spring rolls.

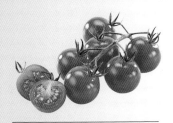

EACH SERVING PROVIDES:

○ Calories 170

○ Protein 3g

○ Carbohydrate 18g
  Fiber 3g

○ Total Fat 10g
  Saturated Fat 2g

○ Sodium 13g

Preparation Time: 20–25 minutes
Serves: 4

EACH SERVING PROVIDES:

○ Calories 135

○ Protein 13g

○ Carbohydrate 2g
  Fiber 0g

○ Total Fat 9g
  Saturated Fat 3g

○ Sodium 430mg

SERVING TIP
As an alternative to muffins, use bagels, rolls, or French bread in this recipe.

Preparation Time: 10 minutes
Serves: 2

POTATO WEDGES

3 large potatoes, cut into wedges
1 tbsp oil
1 tbsp paprika

FOR THE GUACAMOLE
1 avocado, peeled and roughly mashed
½ chili, finely chopped
grated peel and juice of 1 lime
2 tbsp chopped cilantro
salt and freshly ground black pepper, to taste

FOR THE TOMATO SALSA
4oz (125g) cherry tomatoes, roughly chopped
½ small red onion, chopped
1 tbsp chopped fresh parsley

1 Cook the potato wedges in boiling water for 5 minutes. Drain well.

2 Toss together the potato wedges, oil, and paprika, then place on a foil-lined baking sheet and broil under a preheated hot broiler for 4–5 minutes, until crisp and golden.

3 In separate bowls, mix together the ingredients for the two dips. Serve with the potato wedges.

POACHED EGGS & PROSCIUTTO ON ENGLISH MUFFINS

2 English muffins, halved
2 slices prosciutto
(or lean traditional ham)
1 tomato, sliced
2 eggs
salt and freshly ground black pepper, to taste

1 Toast the muffin halves on both sides.

2 Top 2 of the muffin halves with the prosciutto and the tomato. Poach the eggs and place 1 on each of the muffin halves. Season well, top with the other muffin halves, and serve.

SUPER-SIMPLE SMOKED SALMON TARTLETS

9oz (275g) shortcrust pastry, thawed if frozen
4oz (125g) smoked salmon, roughly chopped
1 cup (200ml) low fat crème fraîche
3 eggs, beaten
2 tbsp chopped fresh chives
1 tbsp wholegrain mustard
salt and freshly ground black pepper, to taste

1 Preheat the oven to 400°F/200°C. Roll out the pastry and use to line 8 x 3in (7cm) individual fluted tart pans. Line the pastry cases with foil and fill with dried beans. Bake for 10 minutes. Remove the tart pans from the oven and remove the foil and beans.

2 Mix together the remaining ingredients, then divide among the pastry cases in the tartpans. Return to the oven and bake for 12–15 minutes, until golden and set.

PASTA-STUFFED PEPPERS

4 red peppers, halved, cored,
and seeded (see page 71)
1 cup (125g) small pasta shapes,
such as macaroni, cooked and drained
4 tomatoes, roughly chopped
3¹/₂oz (100g) goat cheese, crumbled
4 scallions, chopped
3 tbsp chopped fresh parsley
salt and freshly ground black pepper, to taste
1 tbsp light vegetable oil

1 Preheat the oven to 400°F/200°C. Place the peppers, cut-side up, on a baking sheet. Bake for 15 minutes.

2 Mix together the pasta, tomatoes, goat cheese, scallions, and parsley. Season to taste and spoon into the pepper halves.

3 Drizzle a little oil over each of the peppers, then return them to the oven and cook for 15–20 minutes, until they are tender.

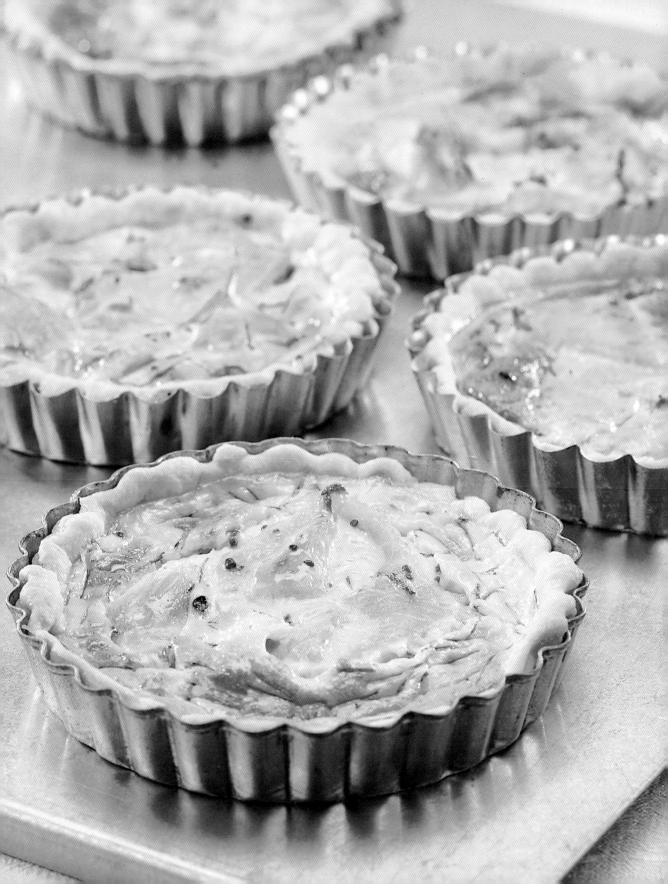

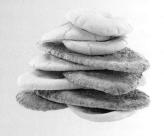

PITA POCKETS STUFFED WITH CHICKEN TIKKA & RAITA

PITA BREADS ARE VERY VERSATILE: RING THE CHANGES WITH

DIFFERENT FILLINGS, SUCH AS THE VARIATIONS BELOW, FOR

PACKED LUNCHES AND PICNICS.

2 tbsp curry paste
6 tbsp plain yogurt
2 boneless, skinless chicken breast halves,
each about 4oz (125g), cubed

FOR THE RAITA
4 tbsp plain yogurt
2 tbsp chopped fresh mint
1 tbsp chopped fresh parsley
1/4 cucumber, grated

TO SERVE
4 pita breads
salad leaves

1 In a bowl, mix together the curry paste and yogurt. Stir in the chicken cubes, coating them well in the mixture. Set aside to marinate for at least 30 minutes.

2 Mix together all the ingredients for the raita and set aside.

3 Place the marinated chicken on a foil-lined baking sheet and broil under a preheated broiler for 5–6 minutes, until cooked through.

4 Sprinkle the pita breads with a little water, then toast for 1–2 minutes, until golden and puffed up. Split open the pita breads and fill them with the salad leaves and chicken tikka. Top with a little raita.

VARIATIONS

Vegetarian Pita Pockets Line the pita breads with lettuce leaves and spoon in equal amounts of chopped cucumber and tomatoes, feta cheese, and pitted black olives.

Pesto Pocket Mix 3 tsp (45g) low fat cream cheese and 1 teaspoon pesto; put in a pita bread with watercress and a few slices of red pepper.

✱ STAR INGREDIENT
Pita bread is a versatile, starchy food that can be served either filled or cut into strips for serving with dips.

EACH SERVING PROVIDES:

○ Calories 334

○ Protein 30g

○ Carbohydrate 47g
    Fiber 2g

○ Total Fat 4g
    Saturated Fat 1g

○ Sodium 571mg

PREPARATION TIP
Prepare the filling in advance, but do not fill the pitta breads until just before serving them.

**Preparation Time: 16–18 minutes, plus 30 minutes marinating
Serves: 4**

Illustrated on page 24

CHICKPEAS WITH SPICY SAUSAGE

EACH SERVING PROVIDES:

○ Calories 354

○ Protein 21g

○ Carbohydrate 37g
  Fiber 9g

○ Total Fat 14g
  Saturated Fat 4g

○ Sodium 657mg

NUTRITION TIP
Sausages like chorizo are high in fat and salt, but quite small amounts provide bean dishes with a good flavour and texture.

Preparation Time: 18 minutes
Serves: 3

1 tsp olive oil
1 onion, sliced
1 garlic clove, crushed
1 tsp hot chili powder
3¹/₂oz (100g) spicy sausage,
such as chorizo, sliced
800g (1lb 10oz) canned chickpeas,
drained and rinsed
1 cup (200g) canned chopped tomatoes
and juice
1 tbsp tomato purée
2 tbsp chopped fresh parsley
salt and freshly ground black pepper, to taste

1 Heat the oil in a medium saucepan. Add the onion, garlic, chili powder, and sausage, and fry gently for 2 minutes.

2 Stir in the remaining ingredients. Bring to a boil, reduce the heat, cover the pan, and simmer for 5 minutes. Taste and adjust the seasoning, if necessary, before turning into a warmed serving dish to serve.

SPINACH TORTILLA

EACH SERVING PROVIDES:

○ Calories 241

○ Protein 13g

○ Carbohydrate 25g
  Fiber 3g

○ Total Fat 10g
  Saturated Fat 3g

○ Sodium 163mg

NUTRITION TIP
Although eggs are high in cholesterol, they have no saturated fat and are a good source of iron and protein.

Preparation Time: 20–25 minutes
Serves: 4 as a light lunch or light supper or 8 as a starter.

2 large potatoes, sliced
1 tbsp olive oil
1 onion, sliced
7 cups (200g) young spinach

3 eggs, beaten
3 tbsp fresh parmesan, grated
¹/₄tsp grated nutmeg
salt and freshly ground black pepper

1 Cook the potatoes in boiling water for 5 minutes, until almost tender. Drain well.

2 Heat the oil in a medium non-stick frying pan. Add the onion and fry for 2–3 minutes. Add the spinach and stir-fry until it has wilted and any moisture has evaporated. Add the potato slices and turn them to combine with the other ingredients.

3 Mix together the remaining ingredients and pour into the pan. Cook over a low heat until almost set. Place under a preheated broiler for 1–2 minutes, until the top is golden and the eggs have set.

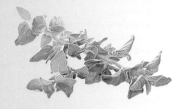

★ STAR INGREDIENT
When highly flavored fresh or dried herbs, such as oregano, are used in recipes, the amount of salt added can be reduced.

EACH SERVING PROVIDES:

○ Calories 276

○ Protein 10g

○ Carbohydrate 40g
Fiber 3g

○ Total Fat 9g
Saturated Fat 2g

○ Sodium 487mg

SERVING TIP
Serve this pizza with plenty of salad, such as a green, leafy salad or a more substantial vegetable salad.

Preparation Time: 40 minutes, plus 30 minutes proving
Serves: 4

FANTASTIC FOUR SEASONS PIZZA

FOR THE PIZZA BASE
1½ cups (180g) bread flour
pinch of salt
1 package (7g) fast-acting yeast
⅔ cup (150ml) warm water
1 tbsp olive oil

FOR THE TOPPING
1 tbsp olive oil
1 onion, sliced
2 garlic cloves, crushed
1 tbsp chopped fresh oregano

¾ cup (400g) canned chopped
tomatoes
1 tbsp tomato purée
⅓ cup (45g) black olives
7oz (200g) canned artichoke hearts,
drained and halved
2 slices prosciutto,
roughly chopped
3 slices salami, chopped
½ red pepper, cored, seeded
and sliced (see page 71)
1½ cups (100g) mushrooms, sliced

1 For the pizza base, put the flour, salt, and yeast in a large bowl and mix together well. Make a well in the center and pour in the warm water and oil. Mix together gently but thoroughly.

2 Turn the dough out on to a lightly floured surface and knead for 5–6 minutes, or until smooth and elastic. Return the dough to a clean, lightly greased bowl, cover with a damp cloth, and set aside in a warm place for 30 minutes, or until doubled in size.

3 Knead the dough again, then roll it out to a 10in (25cm) circle and place on a baking sheet. Preheat the oven to 425°F/220°C.

4 For the topping, heat most of the oil in a non-stick frying pan, add the onion and garlic, and fry gently for 2 minutes. Stir in the oregano, tomatoes, and tomato purée. Bring to a boil, reduce the heat, and simmer for 10 minutes, until thickened.

5 Brush the pizza base with the remaining oil, spoon over the tomato mixture, then scatter the remaining topping ingredients on top. Bake on the bottom rack of the oven for 15–20 minutes, until crisp and golden.

VARIATIONS

Traditional Pizza Add a little cheese, if desired. Choose low fat varieties of Cheddar or mozzarella.

Quick and Easy Pizzas Put the topping on halves of French bread, or on "mini pizzas" made from muffins – ideal for children – and cook them under a preheated broiler.

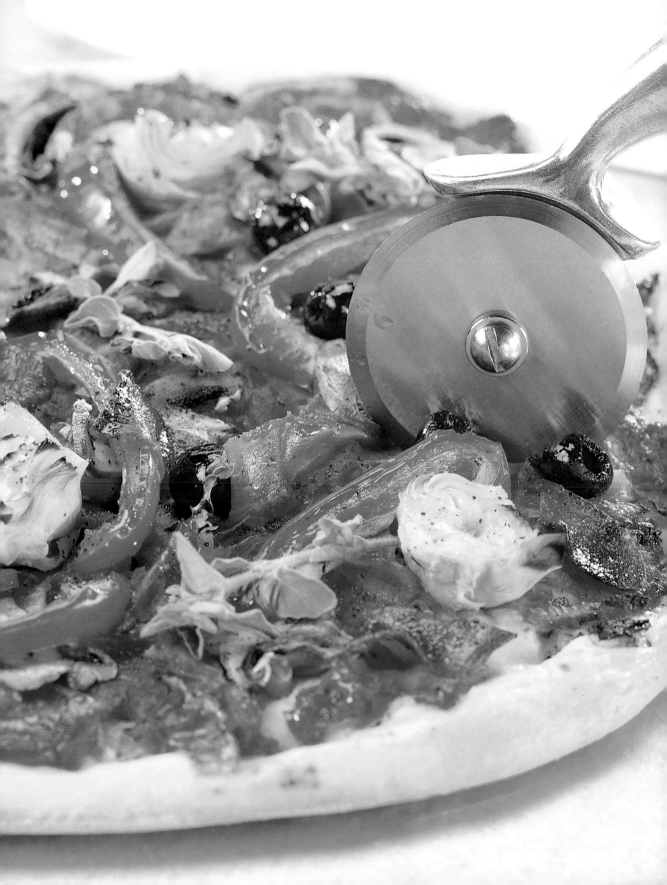

EACH SERVING PROVIDES:

○ Calories 210

○ Protein 7g

○ Carbohydrate 25g
   Fiber 4g

○ Total Fat 9g
   Saturated Fat 2g

○ Sodium 40mg

PREPARATION TIP

Use the minimum amount of oil in preparing the rosti to cut down on fat.

Preparation Time: 25–33 minutes

Serves: 4

ROSTI WITH MIXED MUSHROOMS

2 large potatoes, scrubbed
1 egg, beaten
1 onion, chopped
1 tbsp flour
2 tbsp olive oil
2 garlic cloves, crushed

6 cups (500g) mushrooms, assorted
varieties, including wild if possible
3 tbsp chopped fresh parsley
3 tbsp low-fat crème fraîche
salt and freshly ground
black pepper, to taste

1 Cook the potatoes in their skins in a large pan of boiling water for 10–15 minutes until almost tender. Drain well and skin. Grate the potatoes into a bowl and stir in the egg, onion, and flour. Season well.

2 Divide the potato mixture into 8 balls and form into 'rosti' shapes – flat rounds about 3in (7cm) across.

3 Heat 1 tablespoon of the oil in a non-stick frying pan. Add 4 rosti and fry on high heat for 3–4 minutes on each side, until golden and crisp. Repeat with the remaining rosti. Keep the rosti warm.

4 Heat the remaining oil in a saucepan. Add the garlic and mushrooms and fry gently for 3–4 minutes. Stir through the parsley and crème fraîche, season to taste, and heat through. Serve the rosti topped with the mushroom mixture.

VARIATION

Root Vegetable Rosti Use a mixture of root vegetables such as potato, parsnip, carrot and celeriac as the basis of the rosti.

EACH SERVING PROVIDES:

○ Calories 540

○ Protein 45g

○ Carbohydrate 67g
   Fiber 3g

○ Total Fat 11g
   Saturated Fat 5g

○ Sodium 765mg

Preparation Time: 10 minutes

Serves: 1

STEAK SANDWICH

4oz (125g) sirloin steak, in one piece
½ onion, sliced
1½oz (45g) mushrooms, sliced

½ French loaf, halved lengthwize
large handful arugula leaves
salt and freshly ground black pepper

1 Heat a non-stick frying pan until hot. Put the steak in the pan and fry on high heat for 1–2 minutes, turning it once. Add the onion and mushrooms and fry for a further 1–2 minutes, or until the steak is cooked to your preference.

2 Fill the bread with the steak, mushrooms, and onions, top with the arugula, and season well with salt and pepper.

BLT Bagel with Herb Creme Fraiche

EACH SERVING PROVIDES:

○ Calories 317

○ Protein 20g

○ Carbohydrate 37g
Fiber 2g

○ Total Fat 11g
Saturated Fat 5g

○ Sodium 1321mg

PREPARATION TIP
To reduce the fat content of bacon, choose lean cuts and broil them well.

Preparation Time: 10 minutes
Serves: 1

Illustrated on page 27

---

2 strips lean bacon
1 bagel, halved
1 tomato, sliced
handful of lettuce leaves

1 tbsp low fat crème fraîche
1 tbsp mixed chopped fresh herbs,
such as chives, cilantro,
and parsley
salt and freshly ground black pepper

1 Broil the bacon until crisp under a hot, preheated broiler.

2 Toast the bagel halves on both sides.

3 Layer up the grilled bacon, tomato slices, and lettuce on the bottom half of the bagel.

4 Mix together the crème fraîche, herbs, and seasoning to taste and spoon over the filling. Sandwich together with the other half of the bagel.

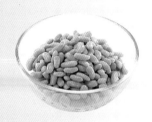

✱ STAR INGREDIENT
Legumes like flageolet beans are good sources of protein and insoluble fibre.

EACH SERVING PROVIDES:

○ Calories 387

○ Protein 28g

○ Carbohydrate 28g
Fiber 9g

○ Total Fat 17g
Saturated Fat 7g

○ Sodium 519mg

Preparation Time: 25–27 minutes
Serves: 3

Lamb & Flageolet Bean Salad

10oz (300g) piece lamb fillet,
trimmed of fat
2 tbsp mixed peppercorns,
roughly crushed
2 tbsp olive oil
1 garlic clove, chopped
1 red onion, cut into wedges

13oz (400g) canned pimentos,
drained and sliced
13oz (400g) canned flageolet beans,
drained and rinsed
2 tbsp balsamic vinegar
fresh herbs, to garnish
(optional)

1 Roll the lamb in the crushed peppercorns to coat well.

2 Heat the oil in a nonstick frying pan until hot. Add the lamb and fry on high heat for 5–6 minutes, turning, until cooked to your preference.

3 Remove the lamb from the pan and set aside.

4 Add the garlic and onion to the pan and fry for 2–3 minutes. Stir in the pimentos, beans, and balsamic vinegar and heat through.

5 Turn the bean salad out of the pan on to a warmed serving dish. Cut the lamb into thin slices and lay them on the bean salad. Garnish with fresh herbs, if desired.

Pan-fried Duck Breasts with Mango Salsa

THE EXOTIC FLAVOR OF THIS SUCCULENT DISH MAKES IT IDEAL

FOR DINNER PARTIES. SERVE IT WITH POTATOES, RICE, OR PASTA,

AND PLENTY OF VEGETABLES.

*4 duck breasts, each about 5oz (150g),
skinned, and trimmed of fat
2 garlic cloves, thinly sliced
1 tbsp paprika
1 tbsp olive oil*

*For the Salsa
1 large mango, peeled and finely chopped
1 red chili, finely chopped
grated peel and juice of 1 lime
2 tbsp chopped cilantro
1 bunch scallions, sliced
salt and freshly ground black pepper, to taste*

1 Make 2 or 3 small cuts in each duck breast and insert a slice of garlic into each cut. Rub each duck breast with a little paprika.

2 Heat the oil in a non-stick frying pan. Add the duck breasts and fry over a medium heat for 5–6 minutes on each side, until cooked.

3 Mix together all the ingredients for the salsa, seasoning it well.

4 Serve the duck breasts with the salsa.

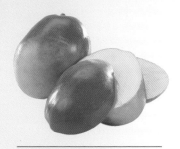

★ STAR INGREDIENT
Mangoes are a good source of beta-carotene, which has antioxidant properties, and which the body can convert to vitamin A.

EACH SERVING PROVIDES:

○ Calories 203

○ Protein 22g

○ Carbohydrate 6g
   Fiber 1g

○ Total Fat 10g
   Saturated Fat 3g

○ Sodium 125mg

PREPARATION TIP
Duck is high in saturated fat; taking off the skin and trimming off all visible fat before cooking will remove most of it.

**Preparation Time: 20–22 minutes
Serves: 4**

MAIN DISHES

Today's healthy eating recommendations focus on starchy foods rather than on planning meals around meat, which was the traditional approach. These recipes offer plenty of scope for mixing meats and vegetables with starchy foods.

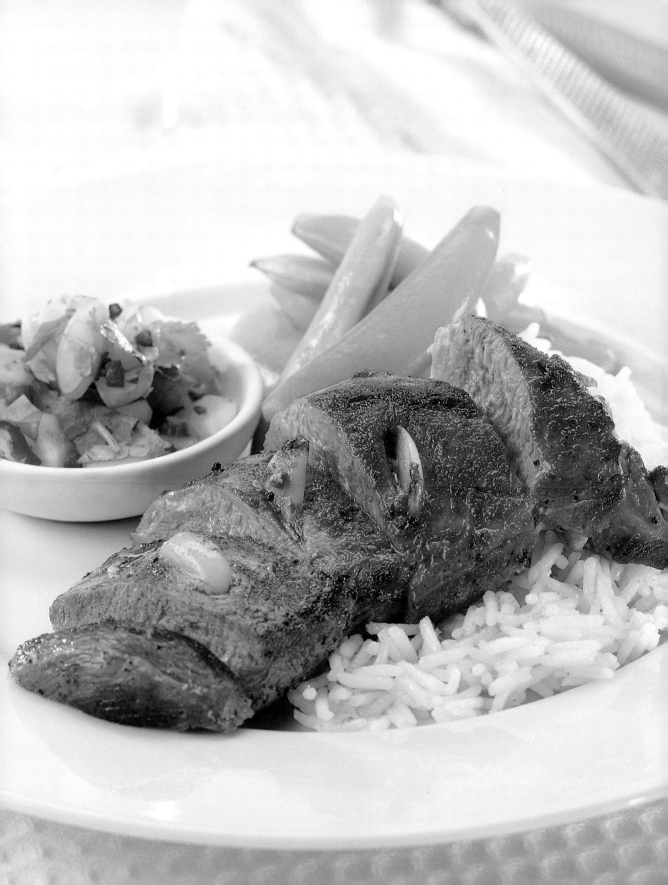

EACH SERVING PROVIDES:

○ Calories 288

○ Protein 44g

○ Carbohydrate 4g
   Fiber 1g

○ Total Fat 10g
   Saturated Fat 4g

○ Sodium 85mg

NUTRITION TIP
For this dish, experiment with other varieties of dried and fresh mushrooms. They are low in calories and contain potassium, niacin, and iron.

Preparation Time: 25 minutes, plus 15 minutes soaking
Serves: 4

CHICKEN WITH MIXED MUSHROOMS & MUSTARD SAUCE

SERVE THIS DISH WITH PLENTY OF BROWN RICE TO SOAK UP THE
DELICIOUSLY PIQUANT AND CREAMY SAUCE, AND WITH A LEAFY
GREEN SALAD ON THE SIDE.

1/2 cup (15g) dried mushrooms, such as porcini
6 tbsp boiling water
1 tbsp olive oil
4 boneless, skinless chicken breast halves,
each about 5oz (150g)
1 small onion, finely chopped
3 cups (200g) fresh mushrooms, sliced
1 cup (200ml) low fat crème fraîche
1 tbsp wholegrain mustard
salt and freshly ground black pepper, to taste

1 Place the dried mushrooms in a small bowl and cover with the boiling water. Let them soak for 15 minutes.

2 Heat half the oil in a non-stick frying pan. Add the chicken breasts and fry over a medium heat for 5–6 minutes on each side, or until they are cooked through. Remove the chicken breasts from the pan, put them on a warmed serving dish, and keep warm.

3 Pour the remaining olive oil into the pan, add the onion, and fry gently for 2 minutes. Add the fresh mushrooms and continue frying gently for 3 minutes.

4 Drain the dried mushrooms, reserving the soaking liquid. Slice the mushrooms and add them to the pan with the soaking liquid. Bring to a boil, reduce the heat, and simmer until the liquid has reduced by half.

5 Stir the crème fraîche and mustard into the pan, bring to a boil, reduce the heat, and simmer gently for 2 minutes. Taste the sauce and season, if necessary. Pour the sauce over the chicken breasts and serve them immediately.

SPINACH & RICOTTA FILLED CHICKEN

4 boneless, skinless chicken breast halves,
each about 5oz (150g)
2 tbsp light vegetable oil
1 small onion, finely sliced
¼ tsp grated nutmeg
4 cups (125g) spinach, washed, drained, and roughly chopped
salt and freshly ground black pepper, to taste
1 cup (200g) ricotta
⅔ cup (150ml) chicken stock

1 Cut a slit in one side of each chicken breast to make a pocket for the stuffing, being careful not to cut right through.

2 Heat half the oil in a non-stick frying pan. Add the onion and fry gently for 2–3 minutes, until softened. Add the nutmeg and spinach and continue to fry for 3–4 minutes, until the spinach is cooked and any moisture has evaporated. Season well, then stir in the ricotta.

3 Stuff the chicken breasts with the spinach mixture and secure the sides with cocktail picks (*see steps 1 and 2, below*). Preheat the oven to 400°F/200°C.

4 Heat the remaining oil in a frying pan. Add the chicken breasts and fry to brown on both sides. Put in an ovenproof dish and add the stock. Bake for 25–30 minutes, until the chicken is cooked through.

STUFFING THE CHICKEN BREASTS

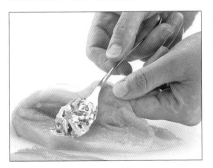 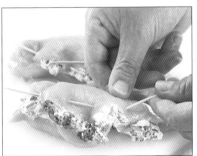

1 Open out each chicken breast pocket and spoon a quarter of the spinach mixture evenly along one side.

2 Lift the uncovered side of the chicken breast over the stuffing and use cocktail sticks to secure the cut sides together.

✳ STAR INGREDIENT
Spinach is a good source of vitamin C and iron. If fresh spinach is not available, use frozen, which has the same nutritional content.

EACH SERVING PROVIDES:

○ Calories 320

○ Protein 47g

○ Carbohydrate 1g
  Fiber 1g

○ Total Fat 14g
  Saturated Fat 5g

○ Sodium 126mg

SERVING TIP
Serve this dish with a carbohydrate food such as potatoes, rice, or pasta, and with a good helping of vegetables.

Preparation Time: 50–55 minutes
Serves: 4

CHICKEN & VEGETABLE PASTA BAKE

A COMPLETE LIGHT MEAL ON ITS OWN, THIS BAKE BECOMES

A MORE SUBSTANTIAL MEAL WHEN SERVED WITH SLICES OF

CRUSTY BREAD AND A SALAD.

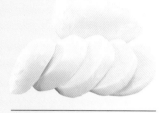

✱ STAR INGREDIENT
Using part-skim mozzarella cheese in cooking reduces a dish's fat content without losing any of the flavor the cheese imparts.

EACH SERVING PROVIDES:

○ Calories 525

○ Protein 13g

○ Carbohydrate 78g
Fiber 5g

○ Total Fat 9g
Saturated Fat 3g

○ Sodium 1655mg

PREPARATION TIP
To turn this dish into a good vegetarian option, replace the chicken with thickly sliced eggplant.

Preparation Time: 20–25 minutes
Serves: 4

1 tbsp light vegetable oil
2 boneless, skinless chicken breast halves,
each about 5oz (150g), chopped
2 zucchini, chopped
1 red pepper, cored, seeded (see page 71), and sliced
2¼ cups (150g) mushrooms, sliced
2 cups (500g) passata (strained tomatoes)
2 tbsp chopped mixed fresh herbs,
such as parsley, oregano, and thyme
salt and freshly ground black pepper, to taste
12oz (375g) dried pasta shapes
4oz (125g) part-skim mozzarella, thinly sliced

1 Heat the oil in a non-stick frying pan. Add the chicken and cook over a medium heat for 3–4 minutes, until browned on both sides.

2 Add the zucchini, pepper slices, and mushrooms, and continue to fry gently for 2–3 minutes.

3 Stir in the tomatoes and herbs, bring to a boil, turn down the heat, and simmer for 2 minutes. Season the sauce well.

4 Meanwhile, cook the pasta in plenty of boiling water for 8–10 minutes, or until al dente. Drain well.

5 Stir the pasta into the sauce, then pour the mixture into a heatproof baking dish. Lay the slices of mozzarella cheese on top.

6 Put the dish under a preheated broiler and cook for 2–3 minutes, until the top is golden and bubbling.

CHICKEN BIRYANI

A STARCHY FOOD LIKE RICE COMBINED WITH VEGETABLES AND

A PROTEIN FOOD SUCH AS CHICKEN MAKES AN IDEAL BASIS

FOR A COMPLETE MEAL – ALL COOKED IN ONE PAN!

1¼ cups (250g) long grain rice

1 tbsp light vegetable oil

2 boneless, skinless chicken breast halves,
each about 5oz (150g), chopped

2 large carrots, sliced

1 large potato, chopped

1 onion, chopped

1 inch (2.5cm) piece fresh ginger, peeled and grated

2 garlic cloves, crushed

½ medium cauliflower, broken into florets

¾ cup (100g) young green beans, halved

2 tbsp medium-strength curry paste

1 tsp turmeric

½ tsp ground cinnamon

½ cup (150g) plain yogurt, plus extra for serving

⅓ cup (60g) golden raisins

3 tbsp chopped cilantro

1 Bring a pan of lightly salted water to a boil, pour in the rice, reduce the heat, and simmer for 8 minutes. Drain well and set aside.

2 Heat the oil in a large, heavy-based saucepan. Add the chicken and fry over a medium heat for 3–4 minutes, turning to brown on all sides.

3 Add the carrots and potato and fry gently for 7–8 minutes, stirring occasionally, until the vegetables are beginning to soften. Add the onion, ginger, garlic, cauliflower, and beans. Stir in the curry paste, turmeric, and cinnamon, and continue to stir-fry for 2–3 minutes. Stir in the yogurt and golden raisins. Pile the rice on top.

4 Cover the pan with a layer of waxed paper or foil, then put on the lid. Cook over a low heat for 10 minutes. Remove from the heat and let it stand, still covered, for 5 minutes.

✳ STAR INGREDIENT
Oils are healthier fat options for cooking than hard fats (*see pages 18–19*), but always use the minimum amount necessary.

EACH SERVING PROVIDES:

○ Calories 361

○ Protein 28g

○ Carbohydrate 47g
Fiber 4g

○ Total Fat 7g
Saturated Fat 1g

○ Sodium 201mg

SERVING TIP
Plain yogurt, served as an extra sauce or condiment, is a good complement to the spicy, piquant flavors of Indian dishes.

Preparation Time: 45–50 minutes, plus 5 minutes standing
Serves: 4

PAELLA

THIS COMBINATION OF SEAFOOD, POULTRY, RICE, AND

VEGETABLES MAKES A SPECTACULAR DISH GUARANTEED

TO IMPRESS FAMILY AND FRIENDS.

1 tbsp olive oil

1 onion, chopped

*1 red pepper, cored, seeded (see page 71),
and sliced*

2 garlic cloves, crushed

2 tsp paprika

*1 boneless, skinless chicken breast half,
about 5oz (50g), chopped*

2 cups (375g) risotto rice

1/3 cup (50ml) dry white wine

2 1/2 cups (600ml) hot chicken stock

1 tbsp tomato purée

few strands saffron

1lb (500g) mixed seafood (see Preparation Tip, left)

2–3 (7oz) plum tomatoes, skinned and chopped

salt and freshly ground black pepper, to taste

4 tbsp chopped fresh parsley, plus extra to garnish

charred lemon and lime quarters, to garnish (optional)

1 Heat the oil in a large, non-stick frying pan. Add the onion, pepper, and garlic, and fry gently for 3–4 minutes, until softened.

2 Stir in the paprika and fry for 1 minute. Add the chicken and fry over a medium heat for 2 minutes, then add the rice. Pour in the wine and simmer until it has been absorbed into the rice.

3 Mix together the chicken stock, tomato purée, and saffron, and add to the rice mixture. Bring to a boil, turn down the heat, cover the pan, and simmer gently for 25 minutes, adding the seafood and plum tomatoes about 7 minutes before the end of the cooking time.

4 Season well and stir in the parsley. Turn the ingredients into a warmed serving dish and serve immediately, garnished with the fresh parsley and the charred lemon and lime quarters, if desired.

✳ STAR INGREDIENT

Shellfish, an essential ingredient of Paella, are low in fat. However, they are high in cholesterol, but cholesterol in food does not cause cholesterol levels (*see pages 12 and 18*) to rise as much as saturated fat or other factors, such as being overweight.

EACH SERVING PROVIDES:

○ Calories 525

○ Protein 33g

○ Carbohydrate 75g
  Fiber 1g

○ Total Fat 7g
  Saturated Fat 1g

○ Sodium 364mg

PREPARATION TIP

Prepared mixed seafood, fresh or frozen, is sold in supermarkets and fish shops. The usual mixture is squid rings and shelled clams, mussels and shrimp; "luxury" mixtures may include scallops and baby octopus.

Preparation Time: 50 minutes
Serves: 4

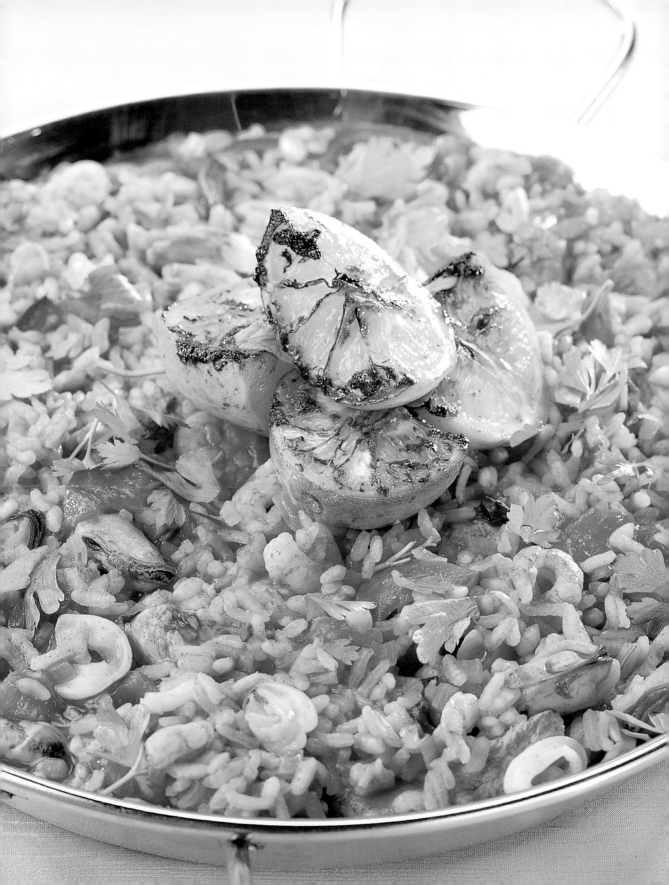

EACH SERVING PROVIDES:

○ Calories 500

○ Protein 42g

○ Carbohydrate 62g
  Fiber 9g

○ Total Fat 11g
  Saturated Fat 4g

○ Sodium 648mg

SERVING TIP
Serve this pie with a mixture
of vegetables. Use either
fresh or frozen, since the
nutrient values are the same.

Preparation Time: 45–50
minutes
Serves: 4

CHICKEN, BUTTER BEAN, TARRAGON & LEEK PIE

THIS VARIATION ON THE TRADITIONAL MEAT PIE WITH

A POTATO, RATHER THAN PASTRY, TOPPING IS AN IDEAL DISH

FOR A FAMILY DINNER.

1 tbsp light vegetable oil
2 boneless, skinless chicken breast halves,
each about 5oz (150g), cubed
2 leeks, sliced
3 cups (250g) mushrooms, sliced
2 tbsp flour
2¹/₂ cups (600ml) low-fat milk
2 tbsp chopped fresh tarragon
¹/₂ cup (60g) sharp cheddar cheese, grated
13oz (400g) canned butter beans, drained and rinsed
salt and freshly ground black pepper, to taste
3 large (750g) starchy potatoes, cooked and mashed
1 tbsp butter

1 Preheat the oven to 400°F/200°C. Heat the oil in a heavy-based saucepan. Add the chicken, leeks, and mushrooms, and stir-fry over a medium heat for 4–5 minutes, until the chicken begins to brown.

2 Stir in the flour and gradually add 2 cups (450ml) of the milk. Gently bring the mixture to a boil, stirring until thickened. Stir in the tarragon, half the cheese, and the butter beans, and season well. Transfer the mixture to an ovenproof dish.

3 Mix together the mashed potatoes, remaining milk, butter, and remaining cheese. Pipe or spoon the potato over the chicken mixture.

4 Transfer the dish to the preheated oven and bake for 20–25 minutes, until the pie is golden and bubbling.

THAI SHRIMP & VEGETABLE CURRY

SERVING TIP
Serve this dish with steamed rice – Thai fragrant rice is particularly appropriate – and a selection of Indian breads.

Preparation Time: 20 minutes
Serves: 4

1 tbsp light vegetable oil
1 onion, chopped
1 red pepper, cored, seeded (see page 71), and chopped
1 yellow pepper, cored, seeded (see page 71), and chopped
6 baby eggplants, quartered or 1 small eggplant, chopped

1½ cups (200g) bamboo shoots
2 tbsp Thai green curry paste
4 kaffir lime leaves
1 stick lemongrass
10oz (300g) large shrimp, thawed if frozen
⅔ cup (150 ml) fish stock
1¾ cup (400ml) coconut milk

1 Heat the oil in a large frying pan. Add the onion, peppers, and eggplants and stir-fry over a high heat for 5–6 minutes, until softened. Add the bamboo shoots, curry paste, kaffir lime leaves, and lemongrass and continue to stir-fry for 2 minutes.

2 Add the shrimp and cook until they have turned pink. Add the stock and coconut milk, bring to a boil, reduce the heat, and simmer for 2 minutes. Turn the curry into a warmed serving dish and serve at once.

PROVENCALE TUNA

NUTRITION TIP
Fresh tuna is an oily fish, containing good amounts of omega 3 fatty acids (*see pages 18–19*). To cut down on fat, use a white fish, such as cod, instead of the tuna.

Preparation Time: 30 minutes
Serves: 4

2 tbsp olive oil
1 large onion, chopped
2 garlic cloves, crushed
1½ cups (400g) canned chopped tomatoes

1 tbsp tomato purée
4 tuna steaks, each about 4oz (125g)
12 pitted black olives
large bunch fresh basil, torn
salt and freshly ground black pepper

1 Heat half the oil in a non-stick frying pan. Add the onion and garlic and fry gently for 3–4 minutes, until softened.

2 Add the tomatoes and tomato purée to the pan, bring to a boil, reduce the heat, cover, and simmer for 5 minutes. Add the tuna steaks, cover, and cook over a low heat for 8–10 minutes.

3 Stir in the olives and basil, being careful not to break the tuna steaks. Heat through, then taste, and season if necessary. Lift the tuna steaks out of the pan and put them on a warmed serving plate or individual plates. Spoon the sauce from the pan over them.

STEAMED FISH PARCELS WITH HORSERADISH & TARTARE SAUCE

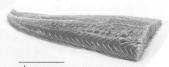

✷ STAR INGREDIENT
Salmon is an oily fish, higher in fat than white fish like cod. However, the fat it contains is a type of polyunsaturated fatty acid that protects against heart disease (*see pages 18–19*).

EACH SERVING PROVIDES:

○ Calories 306

○ Protein 42g

○ Carbohydrate 3g
   Fiber 0g

○ Fat 14g
   Saturated Fat 5g

○ Sodium 180mg

SERVING TIP
Noodles are a good source of carbohydrate, which makes them an excellent accompaniment for this delicately flavored fish dish.

Preparation Time: 20 minutes
Serves: 4

10oz (300g) salmon fillet, skinned and cubed
10oz (300g) cod fillet, skinned and cubed
8 large scallops, deveined
grated peel and juice of 1 lime
1 tbsp butter
salt and freshly ground black pepper

FOR THE SAUCE
6 medium gherkins, finely chopped
1 tbsp capers, drained and chopped
1 cup (200g) low fat crème fraîche
2 tbsp chopped fresh parsley
2 tbsp chopped fresh dill
1 tbsp horseradish sauce
salt and freshly ground black pepper

1 Prepare 4 pieces of baking parchment or aluminium foil, each 10in (25cm) square. Divide the fish and scallops among the papers, drizzle over the lime juice, dot over some butter, and season well. Fold up the pieces of paper to make parcels (*see steps 1 and 2, below*).

2 Put the fish parcels in a steamer over a pan of simmering water, cover, and steam for 5–6 minutes, until cooked.

3 Meanwhile, mix together all the sauce ingredients and pour into a bowl or sauce boat. Serve with the fish parcels, which may be presented intact or opened and the contents arranged on plates.

TO OVEN-STEAM
Put the parcels on a rack in a roasting pan, pour in boiling water (to below the level of the rack), and cook in an oven preheated to 400°F/200°C for about 10 minutes.

MAKING THE PARCELS

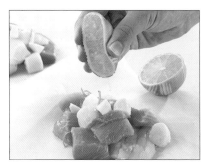

1 Put the ingredients for each fish parcel in the center of each square of paper, leaving plenty of paper all around.

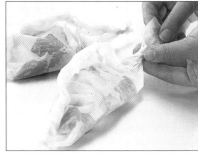

2 Pull up opposite corners of the paper so that a triangular wrapper is formed. Fold the edges and corners together.

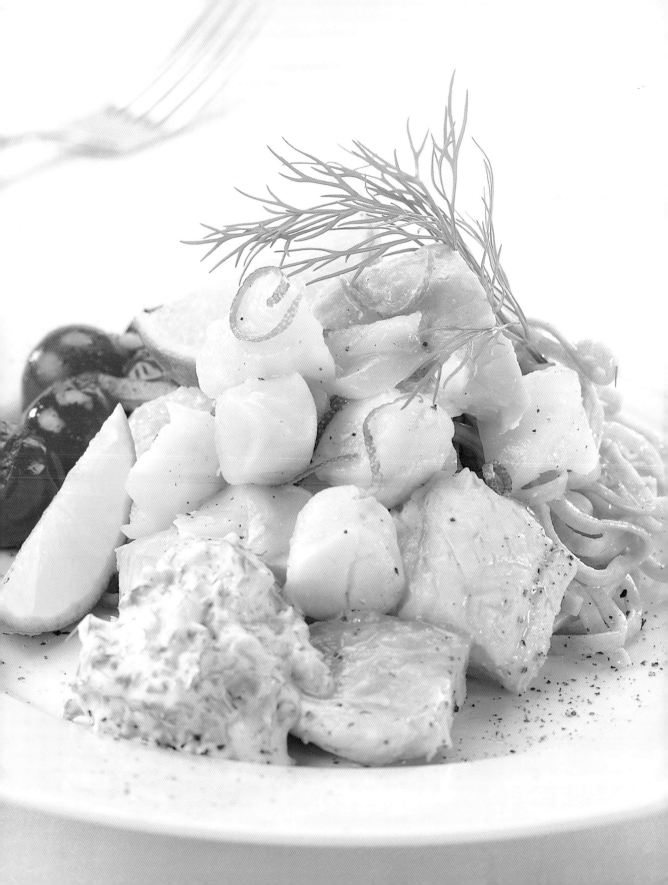

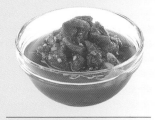

★ STAR INGREDIENT
Canned chopped tomatoes
are a useful storecupboard
ingredient. Their nutritional
value is similar to that of
fresh tomatoes, except for
a lower carotene and
vitamin C content.

EACH SERVING PROVIDES:

○ Calories 214

○ Protein 30g

○ Carbohydrate 12g
  Fiber 3g

○ Total Fat 5g
  Saturated Fat 0g

○ Sodium 92mg

NUTRITION TIP
Replace the pork with
tofu for a good vegetarian
version of this dish.

Preparation Time: 25 minutes
Serves: 4

Illustrated on page 22

Pork & Cilantro Meatballs with Tomato Sauce

THIS IS A SUBSTANTIAL MAIN COURSE DISH. SERVE IT WITH PASTA

OR RICE, AND A TOSSED SALAD OF MIXED LEAVES.

For the Meatballs
1lb (500g) lean ground pork
1 onion, finely chopped
1 garlic clove, crushed
1 tsp dried chili flakes
3 tbsp sun-dried tomato purée
4 tbsp chopped cilantro

For the Sauce
1 onion, chopped
1 garlic clove, crushed
3½ cups (875g) canned chopped tomatoes
⅔ cup (150ml) vegetable stock
2 cups (125g) sun-dried tomatoes
in oil, drained

1 Mix together all the ingredients for the meatballs and form into 12 balls. Place on a baking sheet.

2 Put the meatballs under a preheated broiler and cook them for 6–7 minutes, turning once or twice, until golden and cooked through.

3 Meanwhile, put all the ingredients for the sauce into a saucepan, bring to a boil, reduce the heat, and simmer for 10 minutes. Put half the sauce in a food processor or blender and process until smooth. Return to the pan with the remaining sauce, mix together, and heat through.

4 Add the meatballs to the pan, turning them so that they are well covered in the sauce, and tip the mixture into a warmed serving bowl.

PORK STUFFED WITH BLUE CHEESE & SAGE

EACH SERVING PROVIDES:

○ Calories 400

○ Protein 48g

○ Carbohydrate 0g
   Fiber 0g

○ Total Fat 20g
   Saturated Fat 9g

○ Sodium 606mg

SERVING TIP

Serve with a selection of roast vegetables, such as carrots, zucchini, red onions, and peppers.

Preparation Time: 35–40 minutes
Serves: 4

1lb (500g) pork fillet
4oz (125g) blue cheese, such as stilton or gorgonzola, crumbled
2 tbsp chopped fresh sage

2 tbsp seasoned plain flour
2 tbsp olive oil
2/3 cup (150ml) dry white wine
salt and freshly ground black pepper

1 Cut the pork fillet along its length to make a deep slit, being careful not to cut all the way through. Mix together the cheese and sage, and stuff the mixture into the slit in the pork fillet. Tie the fillet together with string, then roll it in the seasoned flour.

2 Preheat the oven to 400°F/200°C. Heat the oil in a non-stick frying pan. Add the pork and fry gently to brown it all over. Lift the fillet from the pan and put it in an ovenproof dish. Pour the wine into the pan, bring to a boil, reduce the heat, and simmer for 1 minute while scraping up all the sediment in the pan. Pour the liquid over the pork fillet. Bake the fillet for 20–25 minutes, until cooked through.

3 To serve, cut the fillet into slices, then lay the slices on a warmed serving dish. Pour the cooking juices over the fillet.

HERBED PORK STROGANOFF

EACH SERVING PROVIDES:

○ Calories 258

○ Protein 31g

○ Carbohydrate 4g
   Fiber 2g

○ Total Fat 13g
   Saturated Fat 4g

○ Sodium 27mg

SERVING TIP

Serve with a carbohydrate-high food such as rice or noodles and a leafy green salad.

Preparation Time: 25 minutes
Serves: 4

1 tbsp olive oil
1lb (500g) pork tenderloin, sliced
1 onion, chopped
1 garlic clove, crushed
5 cups (375g) mixed mushrooms, such as crimini, porcini, or shiitake, sliced

1 tbsp Dijon mustard
1 tsp paprika
6 tbsp yogurt
8 tbsp low fat crème fraîche
4 tbsp chopped mixed fresh herbs, such as parsley, chives, and sage

1 Heat the oil in a non-stick frying pan. Add the pork slices and fry gently for 3–4 minutes, turning, until browned on both sides.

2 Add the onion and garlic, and continue to stir-fry for 2 minutes. Stir in the mushrooms and continue stir-frying for 3 minutes.

3 Add the remaining ingredients to the pan, bring to a boil, turn down the heat, and simmer for 1 minute, until heated through. Turn into a warmed serving dish and serve immediately.

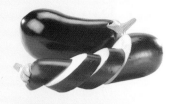

Moroccan Vegetables & Chickpeas on Couscous

2 tbsp light vegetable oil
1 small eggplant, cut into chunks
2 zucchini, cut into chunks
1 carrot, cut into chunks
½ cauliflower, cut into wedges
1 onion, chopped
1 inch (2.5cm) piece fresh ginger,
peeled and grated
2 garlic cloves, crushed
1 tbsp ground cumin
1 tsp chili powder
13oz (400g) canned chopped tomatoes
2 tbsp tomato purée
⅔ cup (150ml) vegetable stock
13oz (400g) canned chickpeas, drained and rinsed
1½ cups (200g) fine green beans, halved
salt and freshly ground black pepper, to taste
1⅓ cups (250g) couscous
1¾ cups (400ml) boiling water
strips of fresh red chili, to garnish
harissa sauce or chili sauce, to serve

1 Heat the oil in a large, heavy-based saucepan. Add the eggplant, zucchini, carrot, cauliflower, onion, ginger, and garlic, and fry gently, stirring, for 3–4 minutes, until the vegetables are beginning to soften.

2 Add the cumin and chili powder, and continue to fry for 1 minute. Add the tomatoes, tomato purée, and vegetable stock, and bring to a boil. Reduce the heat and simmer for 8 minutes, adding the chickpeas and beans halfway through the cooking time. Season well.

3 Meanwhile, put the couscous in a large bowl and pour the boiling water over it. Leave to soak for 8–10 minutes.

4 Serve the vegetables on the couscous, garnished with the red chili strips, and with a little harissa or chili sauce on the side.

✳ STAR INGREDIENT
The eggplant's rich-purple skin and the ability of its flesh to absorb other flavors make it a good basis for vegetarian meals.

EACH SERVING PROVIDES:

○ Calories 339

○ Protein 14g

○ Carbohydrate 58g
   Fiber 9g

○ Total Fat 7g
   Saturated Fat 1g

○ Sodium 230mg

PREPARATION TIP
Eggplants absorb a large amount of oil in cooking; do not be tempted to add more oil than is specified in the recipe.

Preparation Time: 25 minutes, plus 8–10 minutes soaking
Serves: 4

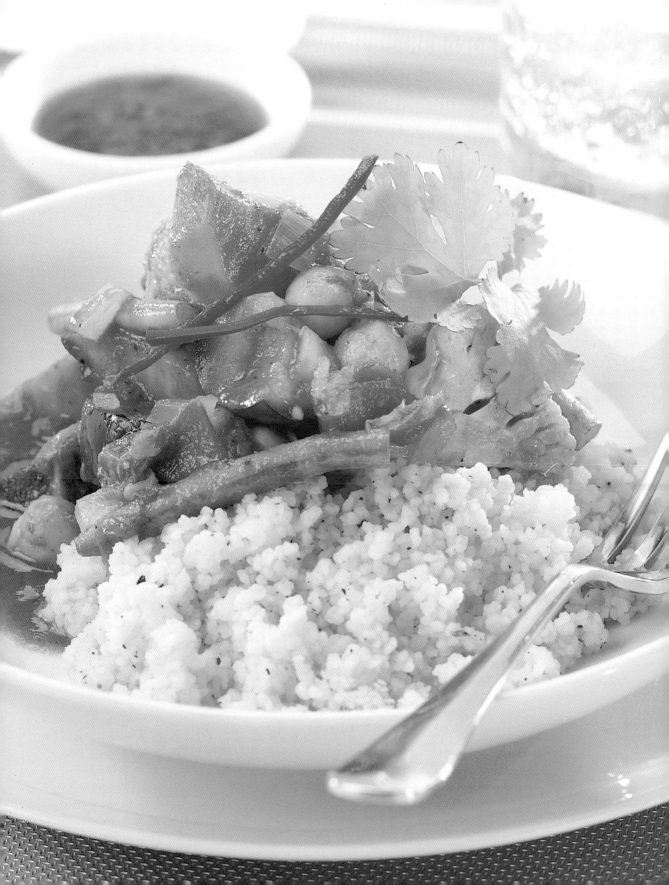

VEGETABLE CASSOULET

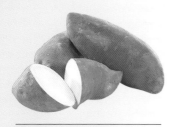

THIS DELICIOUS AND SPLENDIDLY HEALTHY MEAL IS PERFECT FOR

VEGETARIANS AND MAKES A SUBSTANTIAL FAMILY SUPPER.

✳ STAR INGREDIENT
Sweet potatoes are a rich,
low fat source of vitamin E
and antioxidants. Their high
potassium content also makes
them helpful in regulating
high blood pressure.

EACH SERVING PROVIDES:

○ Calories 320

○ Protein 12g

○ Carbohydrate 54g
   Fiber 12g

○ Total Fat 7g
   Saturated Fat 1g

○ Sodium 506mg

PREPARATION TIP
This dish may be frozen,
without the topping, for
up to 3 months. Thaw
completely before adding
the topping and placing
the dish under the broiler.

Preparation Time: 45–50
minutes
Serves: 4

2 tbsp olive oil

2 garlic cloves, crushed

1 large onion, chopped

*1 red pepper, cored, seeded (see page 71),
and chopped*

1 large carrot, chopped

2 sweet potatoes, cubed

1 zucchini, cut into chunks

1 tsp mixed dried herbs

1 bay leaf

13oz (400g) canned chopped tomatoes

1¼ cups (300ml) vegetable stock

2 tbsp tomato purée

*13oz (400g) canned kidney beans,
drained and rinsed*

7oz (200g) fine green beans, halved

1¼ cups (75g) wholewheat breadcrumbs

2 tbsp chopped fresh parsley

1 Heat 1 tablespoon of the oil in a large, heavy-based saucepan. Add the garlic, onion, red pepper, carrot, sweet potatoes, and zucchini. Stir-fry gently for 3–4 minutes, until the vegetables are lightly browned.

2 Add the herbs, bay leaf, tomatoes, stock, tomato purée, and kidney beans. Bring to a boil, reduce the heat, cover, and simmer for 25–30 minutes, until the vegetables are tender. Add the green beans 10 minutes before the end of the cooking time. Transfer to an ovenproof dish.

3 Mix together the breadcrumbs and parsley and scatter over the vegetable mixture. Drizzle the remaining oil over the top, then cook under a preheated broiler until the breadcrumb mixture has browned.

MARINATED TOFU STIR-FRY

EACH SERVING PROVIDES:

○ Calories 147

○ Protein 11g

○ Carbohydrate 12g
   Fiber 5g

○ Total Fat 6g
   Saturated Fat 1g

○ Sodium 21mg

PREPARATION TIP

When marinated, the tofu absorbs the flavors in the marinade, enhancing the flavor of the whole dish.

**Preparation Time: 20–25 minutes, plus 30 minutes marinating
Serves: 4**

1 garlic clove, crushed

2 tbsp soy sauce

1 inch (2.5cm) piece fresh ginger,
peeled and grated

1 tsp dried chili flakes

9oz (275g) tofu, cubed

1 tbsp sesame oil

1 large carrot, grated

1 cup (150g) snow peas, halved

1 red pepper, cored, seeded (see below),
and sliced

3½ cups (275g) mushrooms, sliced

bunch of scallions, chopped

¼ Savoy cabbage, finely shredded

2 cups (200g) beansprouts

❶ Mix together the garlic, soy sauce, ginger, and dried chili flakes in a bowl. Add the tofu and set aside to marinate for about 30 minutes.

❷ Heat the oil in a non-stick frying pan or wok. Lift the tofu from the marinade with a slotted spoon, add to the pan, and stir-fry on a medium heat for 4–5 minutes, until crisp. Remove from the pan and keep warm.

❸ Add the remaining ingredients to the pan, except the beansprouts and marinade, and stir-fry on a medium heat for 2–3 minutes. Add the beansprouts, marinade, and tofu to the pan, heat through, and serve.

PREPARING A PEPPER

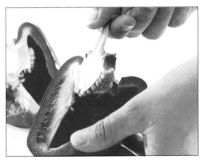 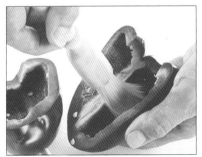

1 Cut the pepper in half. Pull or cut out the stalk and core. Tap each half, cut-side down, to dislodge the seeds.

2 Use a clean pastry brush to brush out any seeds still inside the pepper halves. Discard the seeds and core.

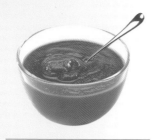

✴ STAR INGREDIENT

Passata is made from puréed Italian tomatoes and is thicker and less smooth than tomato purée. Fat-free and rich in carotenes and vitamin E, passata is an ideal basis for soups, sauces, and casseroles.

EACH SERVING PROVIDES:

○ Calories 567

○ Protein 19g

○ Carbohydrate 82g
    Fiber 7g

○ Total Fat 20g
    Saturated Fat 6g

○ Sodium 146mg

PREPARATION TIP

Toast the pine nuts by dry-roasting them in a non-stick pan. They can be toasted in advance and stored in an airtight container for use in pasta dishes and salads.

Preparation Time: 30 minutes
Serves: 4

CHARRED VEGETABLE PASTA

THIS EASY-TO-MAKE PASTA DISH IS VERY VERSATILE. SERVE IT AT MID-WEEK MEALS, AS A SUBSTANTIAL VEGETARIAN MAIN COURSE, OR AS A MAIN DISH FOR BUFFET-STYLE ENTERTAINING.

2 zucchini, halved lengthways and cut into 3
1 red pepper, cored, seeded (see page 71),
and cut into chunks
1 yellow pepper, cored, seeded (see page 71),
and cut into chunks
1 eggplant, cut into chunks
1 tbsp light vegetable oil
1lb (500g) can passata (puréed tomatoes)
1 cup (200g) low fat cream cheese
salt and freshly ground black pepper, to taste
3 cups (375g) dried pasta shapes

To Garnish
1/2 cup (60g) pine nuts, toasted
handful of fresh basil leaves, torn

1 Put the vegetables on a foil-lined baking sheet and brush with a little of the oil. Broil under a preheated broiler for about 10 minutes, turning them from time to time, until tender and slightly charred.

2 Put the passata and cream cheese in a saucepan and heat gently together, stirring until combined. Stir in the vegetables and season well.

3 Meanwhile, put the pasta into a large pan of boiling water and cook for 8–10 minutes, or until just tender. Drain well. Add the pasta to the vegetable mixture, turning so that the pasta and vegetables are combined. Turn out of the pan into a warmed serving dish, and sprinkle the pine nuts and basil over the top. Serve immediately.

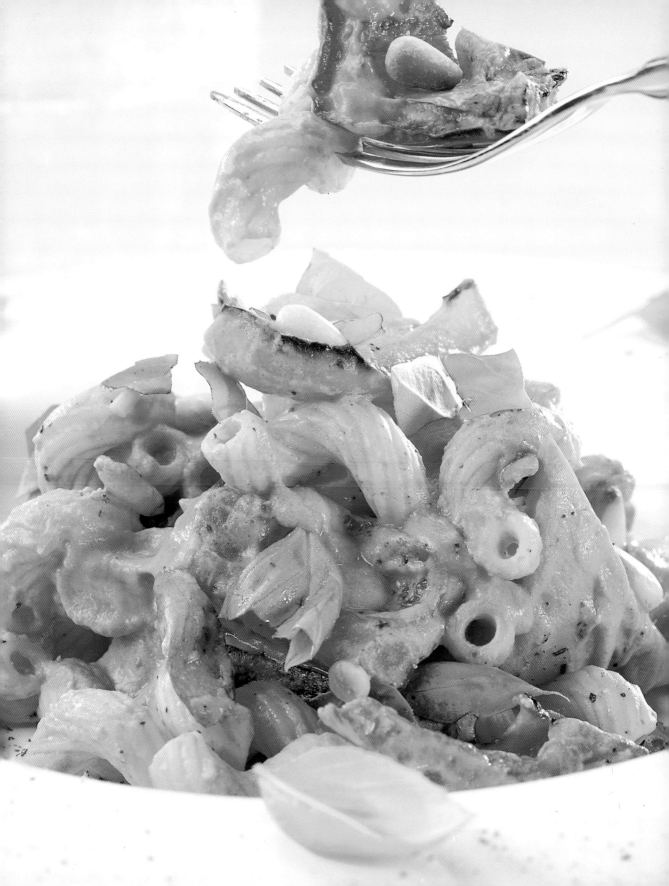

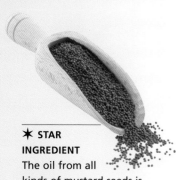

★ STAR INGREDIENT
The oil from all kinds of mustard seeds is high in monounsaturated fat, which is the preferred choice of fat in the diet (*see page 18*).

EACH SERVING PROVIDES:

○ Calories 361

○ Protein 34g

○ Carbohydrate 9g
   Fiber 4g

○ Total Fat 21g
   Saturated Fat 7g

○ Sodium 447mg

PREPARATION TIP
Use beef steaks or chicken breasts instead of lamb in this recipe: both of these meats combine well with the other ingredients.

Preparation Time: 25 minutes
Serves: 4

CORIANDER-CRUSTED LAMB STEAKS WITH EGGPLANTS & RAITA

ENTERTAIN WITH STYLE AND EASE – SERVE THIS DISH WITH PLENTY OF RICE, PASTA, OR POTATOES, AND A GREEN SALAD.

2 tbsp olive oil
1 tbsp black mustard seeds
2 garlic cloves
2 eggplants, cubed
2 red onions, cut into wedges
20 black olives, pitted
4 lean, boneless lamb steaks,
each about 5oz (150g)
1 tbsp ground coriander
salt and freshly ground black pepper,
to taste

FOR THE RAITA
8oz (250g) natural yogurt
¼ cucumber, finely chopped
2 tbsp chopped fresh parsley
2 tbsp chopped fresh mint

1 Heat half the oil in a heavy-based, non-stick frying pan. Add the mustard seeds, garlic, eggplants, and onions, and fry gently for 5–6 minutes, until the eggplants are cooked. Remove from the heat, stir in the olives, and keep warm.

2 Brush the lamb steaks with the remaining oil, rub in the coriander, and season well.

3 Heat a griddle pan or heavy frying pan until hot. Put the lamb steaks in the pan and cook over a high heat for 4–5 minutes on each side.

4 While the lamb steaks are cooking, mix together all the ingredients for the raita.

5 Serve the lamb steaks with the eggplant mixture, and spoon over some raita (or serve the raita separately, if preferred).

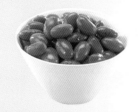

✳ STAR INGREDIENT
Pulses such as lima beans
can help to protect against
heart disease by lowering
cholesterol levels (*see pages
12 and 18*).

EACH SERVING PROVIDES:

○ Calories 462

○ Protein 40g

○ Carbohydrate 42g
  Fiber 10g

○ Total Fat 13g
  Saturated Fat 4g

○ Sodium 690mg

PREPARATION TIP
You can freeze the cooked
and cooled casserole for up
to 3 months.

Preparation Time: 1³/₄–2¹/₄
hours
Serves: 4–6

BEEF, BEER & LIMA BEAN CASSEROLE

THIS IS A HEARTY WINTER CASSEROLE. SERVE IT WITH

POTATOES AND OTHER ROOT VEGETABLES, SUCH

AS CARROTS, PARSNIPS, AND TURNIPS.

1lb (500g) stewing beef, cubed
2 tbsp flour, seasoned with salt and pepper
2 tbsp light vegetable oil
7oz (200g) pearl onions
1¹/₄ cups (300ml) beef stock
12oz (375ml) can beer
2 bay leaves
large sprig thyme
2¹/₂ cups (875g) canned lima beans,
drained and rinsed
3 cups (200g) button mushrooms
salt and freshly ground black pepper,
to taste

1 Toss the meat in the seasoned flour. Heat the oil in a heavy-based frying pan. Add the meat, in batches, and fry over a medium heat until browned on all sides.

2 Remove the meat from the pan (with a slotted spoon so that most of the oil is left behind). Add the onions to the pan and stir-fry gently for 2–3 minutes, until lightly browned.

3 Return the meat to the pan with the stock, stout, and herbs. Bring to a boil, reduce the heat, cover the pan, and simmer gently for 1¹/₂–2 hours, until the meat is tender. Add the beans and mushrooms to the pan halfway through the cooking time.

4 Taste and adjust the seasoning, if necessary, and serve.

PEPPERED BEEF FILLET WITH MASHED POTATO, PEAS & HORSERADISH

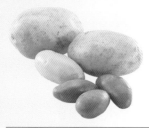

★ STAR INGREDIENT
Potatoes, a staple food in many countries, are a good source of carbohydrate and vitamin C.

EACH SERVING PROVIDES:

○ Calories 446

○ Protein 41g

○ Carbohydrate 33g
Fiber 4g

○ Total Fat 17g
Saturated Fat 9g

○ Sodium 165mg

PREPARATION TIP
Bland mashed potatoes take well to many added flavors. Try chopped fresh herbs, a spice such as nutmeg, or other flavorful ingredients like chopped scallions.

Preparation Time: 25–30 minutes
Serves: 4

THIS IS A STYLISH AND MEMORABLE DISH WHICH IS EXCELLENT FOR DINNER PARTY ENTERTAINING. IT IS ALSO IDEAL FOR A SPECIAL EVENING MEAL AT HOME.

2 tbsp mixed peppercorns, crushed
4 fillet steaks, each about 4oz (125g)
3 large potatoes, roughly chopped
1¼ cups (150g) frozen peas
2 tbsp horseradish sauce
2 tbsp (30g) butter
salt and freshly ground black pepper,
to taste
1 tbsp olive oil

To Garnish
small cubes of red pepper
parsley sprigs

1 Press the peppercorns onto both sides of each steak, then set the steaks aside.

2 For the vegetables, cook the potatoes in boiling water for 12–15 minutes, until tender, adding the peas 2 minutes before the end of the cooking time. Drain well. Add the horseradish sauce, butter, and seasoning to the potatoes, and mash them well together. Keep the mashed potatoes warm while cooking the steaks.

3 Heat the oil in a heavy-based frying pan. Add the steaks and fry over a high heat for 2–3 minutes on each side, or until cooked to your preference.

4 Divide the mashed potato into 4 portions and flatten each to shape it into rounds. Cut the fillet steaks into slices and lay them on top of the potato shapes. Garnish with the red pepper cubes and parsley sprigs and serve immediately.

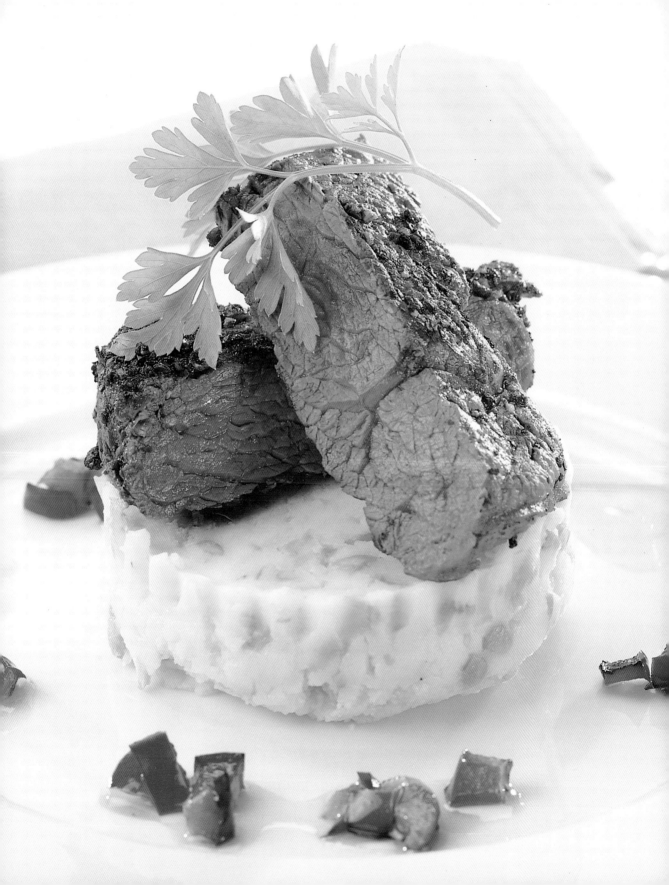

Greek Roast Salad

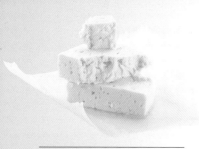

THIS SPLENDID DISH, FULL OF THE FLAVORS OF THE MEDITERRANEAN,

MAY BE SERVED EITHER HOT OR COLD. HAVE PLENTY OF GOOD CRUSTY

BREAD ON THE TABLE FOR EATING WITH IT.

2lb (1kg) zucchini, cut into chunks
2 red onions, cut into wedges
2 red peppers, cored, seeded (see page 71),
and cut into chunks
2 tbsp olive oil
2 sprigs thyme
4 medium (500g) tomatoes, cut into chunks
7oz (200g) feta cheese, cubed
½ cup (60g) black olives
1 tbsp balsamic vinegar
salt and freshly ground black pepper,
to taste

1 Preheat the oven to 400°F/200°C. Spread the zucchini, onions, and peppers out in a roasting pan, drizzle the oil over them, and lay the thyme on top. Bake for 25–30 minutes, until the vegetables are tender and slightly charred.

2 Top with the remaining ingredients and bake for a further 10 minutes. Taste, add seasoning if necessary, and serve.

★ STAR INGREDIENT
Feta cheese has a low fat content compared to other hard cheeses. It is high in sodium, however, a fact that should be remembered when adding salt to recipes containing it.

EACH SERVING PROVIDES:

○ Calories 308

○ Protein 15g

○ Carbohydrate 20g
  Fiber 6g

○ Total Fat 19g
  Saturated Fat 8g

○ Sodium 1076mg

PREPARATION TIP
The vegetables for this dish may be prepared in advance and stored in the refrigerator until needed.

Preparation Time: 50 minutes
Serves: 6

VEGETABLES

Vegetables of all kinds are excellent bases for recipes. Combined with starchy foods like rice and pasta, they make well-balanced meals. Vegetables are good sources of fiber, antioxidant vitamins, and minerals.

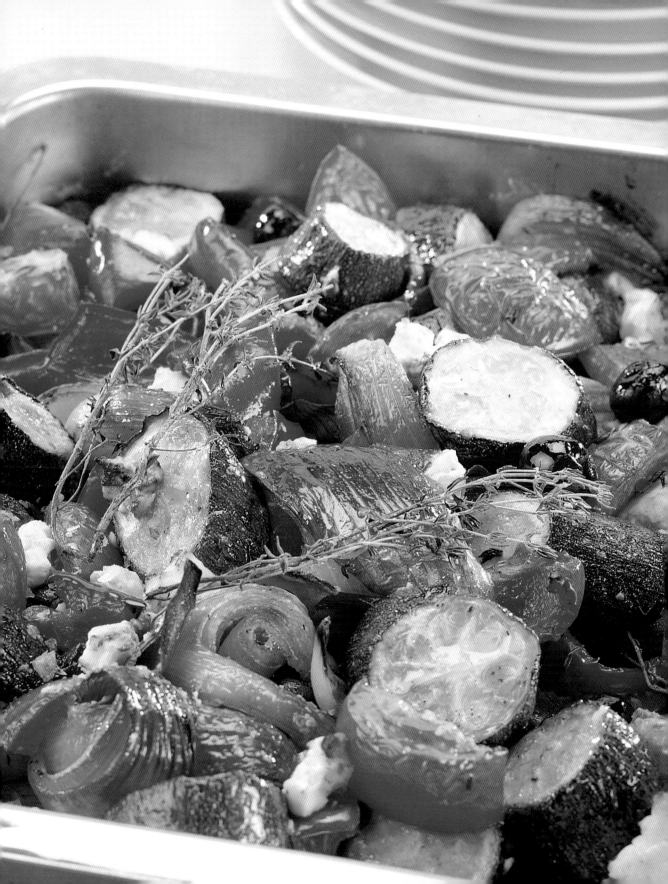

SALADE NICOISE

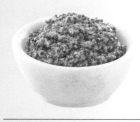

✳ STAR INGREDIENT
Wholegrain mustard gives the dressing for this salad a deliciously nutty texture and a piquant flavor.

EACH SERVING PROVIDES:

○ Calories 188

○ Protein 7g

○ Carbohydrate 16g
  Fiber 4g

○ Total Fat 11g
  Saturated Fat 2g

○ Sodium 445mg

PREPARATION TIP
The ingredients for this salad can be prepared in advance, but the dressing should not be added until just before the salad is served.

Preparation Time: 20 minutes
Serves: 4

SERVE THIS CLASSIC FRENCH SALAD WITH BREAD FOR A DELICIOUS

AND SATISFYING LUNCH. THIS IS ALSO A GOOD DISH FOR SERVING

AS PART OF A BUFFET.

8oz (250g) new potatoes
1 cup (150g) fine green beans, trimmed
2 Cos lettuces, torn into bite-sized pieces
2 hard-boiled eggs, quartered
4 plum tomatoes, quartered
¼ cucumber, chopped into bite-sized pieces
20 black olives, pitted

FOR THE DRESSING
1 tbsp wholegrain mustard
2 tbsp olive oil
1 tbsp white wine vinegar
1 tsp sugar
salt and freshly ground black pepper,
to taste

1 Cook the potatoes in boiling water until tender, adding the beans 5 minutes before the end of the cooking time. Drain and refresh under cold, running water. Drain well.

2 Arrange the lettuce pieces in a large salad bowl or serving dish. Toss together the potatoes, beans, eggs, tomatoes, cucumber, and olives, and spoon them over the lettuce in the bowl.

3 Whisk together the dressing ingredients and season well. Drizzle the dressing over the salad and serve.

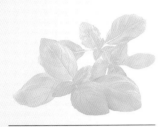

✴ STAR INGREDIENT
Fresh basil's distinctive taste added to a recipe allows the amount of salt to be kept to a minimum.

EACH SERVING PROVIDES:

○ Calories 534

○ Protein 10g

○ Carbohydrate 50g
Fiber 3g

○ Total Fat 12g
Saturated Fat 1g

○ Sodium 12mg

PREPARATION TIP
This is a good recipe for using up leftover cooked pasta.

Preparation Time: 25 minutes
Serves: 4

EACH SERVING PROVIDES:

○ Calories 119

○ Protein 5g

○ Carbohydrate 13g
Fiber 3g

○ Total Fat 5g
Saturated Fat 1g

○ Sodium 41mg

PREPARATION TIP
Using a food processor to prepare the vegetables makes this salad very quick to make.

Preparation Time: 20 minutes
Serves: 6

HERBED PASTA SALAD

2 cups (250g) pasta shapes
2 zucchini, thinly sliced
⅔ cup (150g) cherry tomatoes, halved
2 tbsp pine nuts, toasted
salt and freshly ground black pepper, to taste

FOR THE DRESSING
2 tbsp olive oil
1 tbsp capers, drained
2 tbsp fresh parsley
2 tbsp fresh basil
1 garlic clove
grated peel and juice of 1 lime

1 First, make the dressing. Put all the ingredients in a blender or food processor and process until combined.

2 Cook the pasta in plenty of boiling water until it is tender, but still firm. Drain well.

3 In a large bowl, gently toss together all the salad ingredients, including the pasta. Pour the dressing over the ingredients, tossing to distribute thoroughly. Transfer the salad to a serving dish.

HEALTHY COLESLAW

½ small white cabbage, finely shredded
2 carrots, grated
1 bunch scallions, sliced
⅓ cup (75g) ready-to-eat dried apricots
3 tbsp pumpkin seeds, toasted
*4 tbsp mixed chopped fresh herbs,
such as parsley and mint*
⅔ cup (150m) plain yogurt
2 tbsp low-fat crème fraîche
salt and freshly ground black pepper, to taste

Put all the ingredients in a large salad bowl, turning them together to mix. Taste and adjust the seasoning, if necessary.

EACH SERVING PROVIDES:

○ Calories 382

○ Protein 8g

○ Carbohydrate 60g
Fiber 2g

○ Total Fat 13g
Saturated Fat 2g

○ Sodium 109mg

SERVING TIP
This is an ideal accompaniment for fish and meat dishes.

Preparation Time: 15 minutes, plus 20–25 minutes soaking
Serves: 6

TABBOULEH

1¹/₃ cups (250g) bulgar wheat
1¹/₄ cups (300ml) boiling water
²/₃ cup (150g) cherry tomatoes, quartered
¹/₄ cucumber, finely chopped
6 scallions, finely chopped
4 tbsp chopped fresh parsley
4 tbsp chopped fresh mint
grated peel and juice of 1 lemon
1 tbsp olive oil
salt and freshly ground black pepper,
to taste

1 Put the bulgar wheat in a bowl and pour the boiling water over it. Set aside to soak for 20–25 minutes, until the grains are tender. Pour the bulgar through a strainer to drain off any excess water, then pour it into a serving bowl.

2 Mix together the remaining ingredients and stir them into the bulgar, combining them thoroughly. Taste and adjust the seasoning, if necessary, then serve.

EACH SERVING PROVIDES:

○ Calories 209

○ Protein 3g

○ Carbohydrate 28g
Fiber 2g

○ Total Fat 10g
Saturated Fat 2g

○ Sodium 102mg

PREPARATION TIP
Add the minimum of salt to this recipe; the balsamic vinegar should provide most of the extra flavoring it needs.

Preparation Time: 25 minutes
Serves: 4–6

DELICIOUS POTATO SALAD

2lb (1kg) new potatoes
6 scallions, chopped
8 sun-dried tomatoes in oil,
drained and sliced,
plus 3 tablespoons of the oil
2 tbsp balsamic vinegar
handful of fresh basil leaves, torn
salt and freshly ground black pepper,
to taste

1 Cook the potatoes in boiling water until tender but still firm. Pour through a colander to drain well.

2 Toss the warm potatoes and the remaining ingredients together in a large serving bowl. Taste and adjust the seasoning, if necessary. Serve the salad warm or cold.

PESTO VEGETABLE KEBABS

FOR THE MARINADE
grated peel and juice of ¹/₂ lemon
1 tbsp wholegrain mustard
2 tbsp pesto
1 tbsp olive oil

FOR THE KEBABS
1lb (500g) assorted small vegetables,
such as cherry tomatoes, zucchini wedges,
button mushrooms, and eggplant cubes

1 Combine all the marinade ingredients together in a small bowl. Thread the vegetables on to kebab sticks and put the sticks on a large, flat plate. Pour the marinade over the vegetables and set aside to marinate for 30 minutes, turning the kebabs once or twice.

2 Cook the kebabs under a preheated broiler for 5–6 minutes, turning occasionally, until the vegetables are tender.

MEDITERRANEAN BREAD SALAD

¹/₂ French bread loaf, torn into
bite-sized pieces
1/3 cup (45g) pine nuts
6 plum tomatoes, cut into chunks
¹/₂ cucumber, cut into chunks
2 tbsp capers, drained
1 red onion, finely sliced
2 tbsp chopped fresh parsley
12 black olives
2 tbsp olive oil
1 tbsp red wine vinegar
salt and freshly ground black pepper,

1 Place the pieces of bread in a single layer on a baking sheet and toast under a preheated broiler, turning the pieces, for 1–2 minutes, until golden all over.

2 Put the pine nuts in a small pan and cook over high heat for 1–2 minutes, until lightly toasted.

3 Put the remaining ingredients in a large bowl, add the bread and pine nuts, and toss together gently. Set the salad aside for 30 minutes to allow the flavors to develop before serving.

EACH SERVING PROVIDES:

○ Calories 175

○ Protein 7g

○ Carbohydrate 7g
 Fiber 5g

○ Total Fat 13g
 Saturated Fat 3g

○ Sodium 133mg

Preparation Time: 15 minutes, plus 30 minutes marinating
Serves: 4

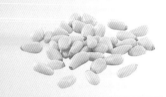

★ STAR INGREDIENT
Pine nuts, with a similar nutritional content to other nuts, are very high in vitamin E.

EACH SERVING PROVIDES:

○ Calories 282

○ Protein 7g

○ Carbohydrate 30g
 Fiber 3g

○ Total Fat 16g
 Saturated Fat 2g

○ Sodium 444mg

Preparation Time: 15 minutes, plus 30 minutes marinating
Serves: 4

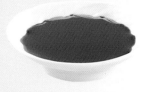

✱ STAR INGREDIENT
Soy sauce is high in sodium.
As it has a strong flavor, it
can be used sparingly.

EACH SERVING PROVIDES:

○ Calories 233

○ Protein 8g

○ Carbohydrate 9g
    Fiber 5g

○ Total Fat 18g
    Saturated Fat 2g

○ Sodium 6mg

Preparation Time: 15 minutes
Serves: 4

Illustrated right

SAUTEED CABBAGE WITH TOASTED SEEDS

1 green cabbage, shredded
1 tbsp light vegetable oil
2 garlic cloves, crushed
1 tbsp mustard seeds
³/₄ cup (125g) mixed seeds,
such as sunflower, pumpkin, and sesame
2 tbsp dark soy sauce

1 Cook the cabbage in boiling water for 5–6 minutes, until almost tender. Pour into a colander and drain well.

2 Meanwhile, heat the oil in a deep-sided, heavy-bottomed frying pan. Add the garlic and fry over a medium heat for 1 minute. Add the mustard seeds and the mixed seeds and continue to cook on medium heat for 2 minutes, so that the seeds brown but do not burn.

3 Take the pan off the heat, add the cabbage, and turn the ingredients with two spoons to mix them well. Sprinkle the soy sauce over the ingredients, return the pan to the heat, and warm through.

EACH SERVING PROVIDES:

○ Calories 151

○ Protein 2g

○ Carbohydrate 7g
    Fiber 6g

○ Total Fat 7g
    Saturated Fat 4g

○ Sodium 70mg

Preparation Time: 45 minutes
Serves: 6

ORANGE & HONEY PARSNIPS

1¹/₂lb (750g) parsnips, peeled and halved
3 tbsp (45g) butter
2 tbsp honey
grated peel and juice of 1 orange
salt and freshly ground black pepper,
to taste

1 Preheat the oven to 400°F/200°C. Partially cook the parsnips in boiling water for 5 minutes. Drain well.

2 Melt the butter in a saucepan and stir in the honey, and the grated orange peel and juice. Season well.

3 Coat the parsnips in the orange mixture and spread out in a roasting pan. Roast in the oven for 25–30 minutes, until golden and crisp.

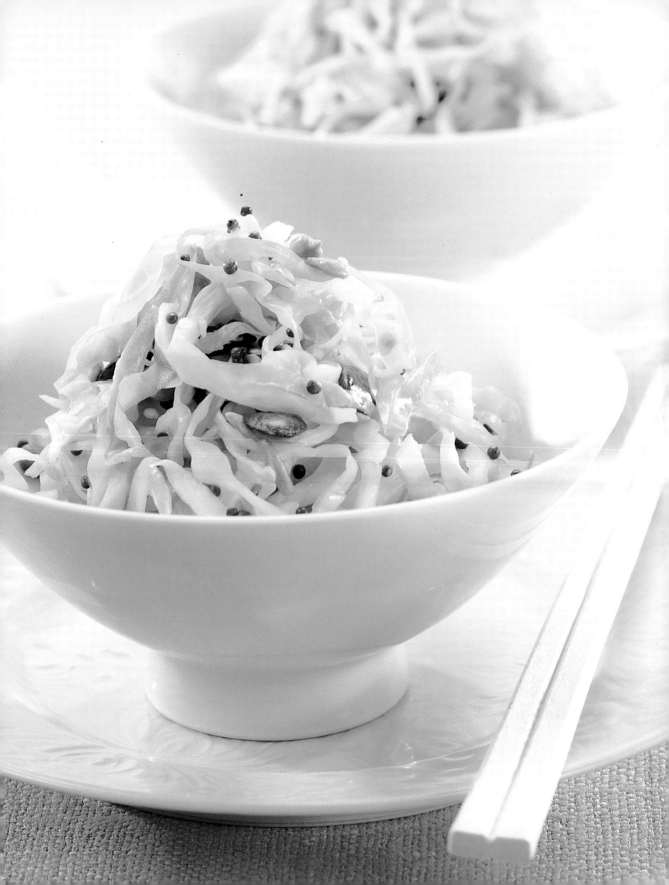

EACH SERVING PROVIDES:

○ Calories 276

○ Protein 20g

○ Carbohydrate 28g
Fiber 5g

○ Total Fat 10g
Saturated Fat 3g

○ Sodium 569mg

**Preparation Time: 40 minutes
Serves: 6**

WARM LENTIL SALAD

1¼ cups (300g) lentils
1½ cups (600ml) vegetable stock
2 tbsp olive oil
2 garlic cloves, sliced
1 red onion, sliced
1 red pepper, cored, seeded (see page 71), and chopped
3 strips lean bacon, chopped
¾ cup (100g) feta cheese, crumbled
1 tbsp balsamic vinegar
2 tbsp chopped fresh parsley
salt and freshly ground black pepper, to taste

1 Put the lentils in a large pan and pour in the stock. Bring to a boil, turn down the heat, cover, and simmer for 20–25 minutes, until the lentils are tender. Drain well.

2 Heat the oil in a frying pan. Add the garlic, onion, and pepper, and stir-fry over a medium heat for 3–4 minutes, until the vegetables have softened. Add the bacon and continue to stir-fry for 3 minutes.

3 Add the lentils and the remaining ingredients to the frying pan and mix well to combine. Taste and adjust the seasoning, if necessary. Turn the salad into a warmed serving dish and serve at once.

EACH SERVING PROVIDES:

○ Calories 90

○ Protein 2g

○ Carbohydrate 7g
Fiber 2g

○ Total Fat 6g
Saturated Fat 1g

○ Sodium 30mg

SERVING TIP
Serve the tomatoes with pasta
to make a complete meal.

**Preparation Time: 45 minutes
Serves: 4**

OVEN-ROASTED TOMATOES

4 cups (1kg) cherry tomatoes
2 tbsp olive oil
2 garlic cloves
handful of fresh basil, torn
salt and freshly ground black pepper, to taste

1 Preheat the oven to 350°F/180°C. Place the tomatoes in an ovenproof dish, drizzle the oil over them, and add the garlic. Season well.

2 Roast in the oven for 35–40 minutes, until the tomatoes are tender and beginning to brown.

3 Transfer to a serving dish. Sprinkle the basil over the tomatoes, and turn them gently so that the basil is thoroughly mixed in.

EACH SERVING PROVIDES:

○ Calories 45

○ Protein 1g

○ Carbohydrate 2g
  Fiber 3g

○ Total Fat 4g
  Saturated Fat 0g

○ Sodium 11mg

Preparation Time: 50 minutes
Serves: 6

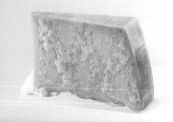

★ STAR INGREDIENT
Parmesan is high in fat, but because of its strong flavor, it can be used sparingly.

EACH SERVING PROVIDES:

○ Calories 160

○ Protein 9g

○ Carbohydrate 5g
  Fiber 4g

○ Total Fat 12g
  Saturated Fat 5g

○ Sodium 173mg

SERVING TIP
Served with warm, crusty bread, this makes a satisfying vegetarian meal.

Preparation Time: 1 hour
Serves: 4

ROAST FENNEL

*4 heads of fennel, trimmed and
cut into quarters lengthways
grated peel and juice of 2 lemons
2 tbsp olive oil
2 tsp cumin seeds
salt and freshly ground black pepper,
to taste*

1 Preheat the oven to 400°F/200°C/400°F. Put all the ingredients in a non-metallic ovenproof dish and toss together well. Season to taste, if necessary.

2 Roast for 35–40 minutes, or until the fennel is golden and tender.

EGGPLANT PARMIGIANA

*3 large eggplants,
cut lengthways into thick slices
2 tbsp olive oil
3 cups (750g) canned chopped tomatoes
handful mixed fresh herbs,
such as basil, parsley, and thyme, roughly chopped
2 garlic cloves, crushed
salt and freshly ground black pepper, to taste
5oz (150g) part-skim mozzarella cheese, grated
2 tbsp freshly grated parmesan cheese*

1 Preheat the oven to 400°F/200°C. Put the eggplant slices in a single layer on a baking sheet and brush them lightly with the oil. Bake in the oven for 20 minutes until the slices are starting to brown.

2 Meanwhile, put the tomatoes, herbs, and garlic in a small saucepan and simmer for 10 minutes. Season well.

3 Layer the eggplant slices and the tomato sauce in an ovenproof dish, finishing with a layer of the sauce. Scatter the mozzarella and parmesan cheeses over the top.

4 Put the dish in the oven and bake for 25–30 minutes, until the top is golden and bubbling. Serve immediately.

Broiled Sweet Potatoes

3 large (625g) sweet potatoes, scrubbed
2 tbsp olive oil
salt and freshly ground black pepper, to taste
2 tbsp chopped cilantro, to garnish

1 Place the potatoes in a pan of boiling water and simmer for about 20 minutes, until almost tender. Drain well.

2 Cut the potatoes into slices approximately ½in (1cm) thick. Brush the slices with the olive oil and season well. Cook under a preheated broiler for 2–3 minutes on each side until golden. Serve in a warmed serving dish, garnished with the cilantro.

Zucchini & Mushroom Bake

1 tbsp olive oil
2 garlic cloves, crushed
1 onion, sliced
2 large zucchini, sliced
2¾ cups (200g) mushrooms, quartered
1½ cups (400g) canned chopped tomatoes
2 tbsp tomato purée
1 tsp dried mixed herbs
salt and freshly ground black pepper, to taste
1 cup (60g) fresh granary breadcrumbs
1½ cups (60g) sharp cheddar cheese, grated

1 Heat the oil in a non-stick frying pan. Add the garlic, onion, and zucchini, and fry gently for 4–5 minutes, until the vegetables are softened and beginning to brown.

2 Add the mushrooms to the pan and continue to fry for 2 minutes. Pour in the tomatoes and their juice, and add the tomato purée. Add the herbs. Simmer for 5 minutes, uncovered. Season to taste.

3 Transfer the mixture to an ovenproof dish. Mix together the breadcrumbs and cheese and sprinkle on top of the vegetables.

4 Put the dish under a preheated broiler for 1–2 minutes, until the top is golden and bubbling.

EACH SERVING PROVIDES:

- Calories 185
- Protein 2g
- Carbohydrate 33g
  Fiber 4g
- Total Fat 6g
  Saturated Fat 1g
- Sodium 62mg

Preparation Time: 35 minutes
Serves: 4

✳ STAR INGREDIENT
The firm yet tender texture and delicious flavor of mushrooms make them excellent additions to vegetarian dishes.

EACH SERVING PROVIDES:

- Calories 194
- Protein 10g
- Carbohydrate 20g
  Fiber 4g
- Total Fat 9g
  Saturated Fat 4g
- Sodium 280mg

PREPARATION TIP
Granary bread's nutty flavor and coarse texture make it an ideal topping, but any fresh breadcrumbs may be used for this dish.

Preparation Time: 25 minutes
Serves: 4

SERVING TIP
Also known as celery root, celeriac is much more stylish than simple mashed potatoes. This is a good dish to serve at a dinner party.

Preparation Time: 25 minutes
Serves: 4

PUREED CELERIAC

2 large potatoes,
peeled and chopped
2³/₄ cups (375g) celeriac,
peeled and chopped
²/₃ cup (150ml) low fat milk
4 tbsp (60g) butter
pinch of nutmeg
salt and freshly ground black pepper,
to taste

1 Cook the potatoes and celeriac together in boiling water for 12–15 minutes, until tender. Drain well.

2 Add the milk, butter, and nutmeg to the potatoes and celeriac, stirring them in with a fork. Mash all the ingredients together to form a smooth mixture. Season well and serve.

✱ **STAR INGREDIENT**
Coriander is a member of the carrot family. Its leaves, known as cilantro, are used as an herb and its seeds as a spice. Both give their distinctive flavors to this dish.

Preparation Time: 25 minutes
Serves: 4

MASHED SWEET POTATO & CILANTRO

4 large (1kg) sweet potatoes,
peeled and chopped
4 tbsp (60g) butter
1 onion, finely chopped
1 tsp ground coriander
1 tbsp black mustard seeds
3 tbsp chopped cilantro
salt and freshly ground black pepper,
to taste

1 Cook the sweet potatoes in boiling water for 10–12 minutes, or until tender. Drain well.

2 Meanwhile, heat the butter in a small pan. Add the onion and fry gently for 3–4 minutes. Add the ground coriander and mustard seeds, and continue to fry for a further minute.

3 Mash the sweet potatoes and combine with the onion mixture and the cilantro. Season well.

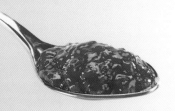

SUMMER FRUIT SORBET

THIS REFRESHING SORBET MADE FROM FROZEN SUMMER FRUITS IS

A REAL TREAT. EASY TO MAKE AND EVEN EASIER TO EAT,

IT WILL SATISFY ANY SWEET TOOTH.

4 cups (500g) frozen mixed summer fruits,
such as raspberries, blueberries,
and strawberries
grated peel and juice of
1 large orange
1 tbsp raspberry jam
mint sprigs, to decorate
fresh berry fruits, to serve

1 Put a food-processor bowl or blender jug in the refrigerator for a few minutes to make sure that it is really cold. Place all the ingredients in the cooled food-processor bowl and process until smooth.

2 Scoop out the sorbet and serve immediately, decorated with sprigs of fresh mint. Serve fresh berry fruits with the sorbet.

VARIATION

Single Fruit Sorbets Replace the mixed frozen fruits with a single frozen fruit, such as raspberries, black raspberries, or strawberries. Match the jam to the fruit.

★ STAR INGREDIENT
You can use ordinary jam for this recipe, rather than the sugar-free kind. The amount of sugar is so small that it will not affect diabetes control.

EACH SERVING PROVIDES:

○ Calories 72

○ Protein 2g

○ Carbohydrate 17g
  Fiber 2g

○ Total Fat 0g
  Saturated Fat 0g

○ Sodium 5mg

PREPARATION TIP
Once made, the sorbet may be stored in the freezer. It will keep for 3 months.

Preparation Time: 15 minutes
Serves: 4

DESSERTS

Fruits make perfect bases for many kinds of cool and hot desserts. They are both fat-free and good sources of antioxidant vitamins, especially vitamin C. These recipes include a great variety of fruits, both familiar and exotic.

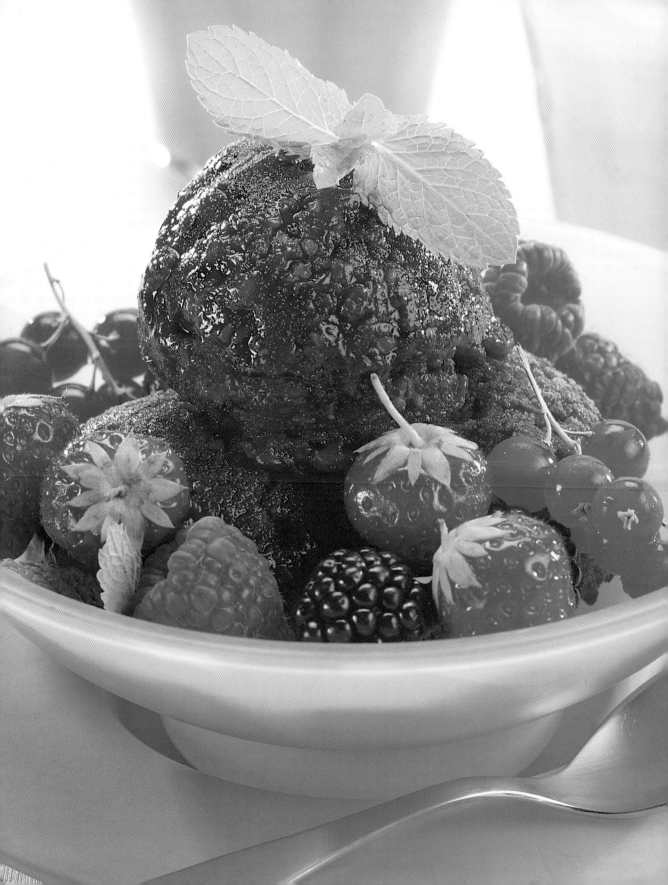

Mango & Lime Sorbet

¼ cup (60g) sugar
⅔ cup (150ml) boiling water
*3 large, ripe mangoes, peeled
and the flesh cut into cubes*
grated peel and juice of 4 limes

1 Tip the sugar into the boiling water in a heavy-bottomed saucepan and stir until dissolved. Cool and chill the syrup in the refrigerator.

2 Put the mango flesh and grated lime peel and juice in a food processor or blender and blend until smooth.

3 Pour the chilled syrup into the food processor and blend for a further 30 seconds.

4 Transfer the mixture to ice trays and freeze for 1½ hours. Remove from the freezer and whisk to remove any ice crystals. Return the ice trays to the freezer and freeze the mixture until solid, whisking it every hour to prevent ice crystals from forming.

EACH SERVING PROVIDES:

○ Calories 116

○ Protein 0g

○ Carbohydrate 30g
   Fiber 3g

○ Total Fat 0g
   Saturated Fat 0g

○ Sodium 32mg

SERVING TIP

Serve scoops of the sorbet in tall glasses for an elegant dinner party dessert.

Preparation Time: 10 minutes, plus 4 hours cooling and freezing
Serves: 4

Blueberry Meringue Ice Cream

THIS DELICIOUS BLEND OF SUMMER BERRIES, CREME FRAICHE, AND CRUNCHY CRUSHED BAKED MERINGUES IS LOWER IN FAT THAN MOST DAIRY ICE CREAMS.

1¾ cups (200g) blueberries
4 tbsp powdered sugar
2 cups (500ml) low fat crème fraîche
2oz (60g) baked meringues, lightly crushed

1 In a food processor or blender, mix together the blueberries, icing sugar, and crème fraîche, until just blended.

2 Stir the crushed meringues through the mixture, then transfer it to ice trays. Freeze for 2–3 hours, until almost frozen but still soft enough to scoop out. Serve at once or store in the freezer.

EACH SERVING PROVIDES:

○ Calories 172

○ Protein 2g

○ Carbohydrate 24g
   Fiber 1g

○ Total Fat 8g
   Saturated Fat 5g

○ Sodium 30mg

SERVING TIP

If the ice cream has been made ahead of time, remember to take it out of the freezer and put it in the refrigerator 30 minutes before it is to be served.

Preparation Time: 10 minutes, plus 2 hours freezing
Serves: 6

CHOCOLATE, CINNAMON & PEAR TART

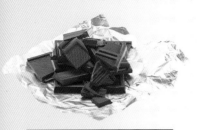

★ STAR INGREDIENT
Choose semisweet chocolate with a high cocoa solid content for all dessert making. Chocolate that is labelled "suitable for diabetics" is just as high in fat and calories as standard kinds of chocolate.

EACH SERVING PROVIDES:
○ Calories 293

○ Protein 5g

○ Carbohydrate 28g
  Fiber 2g

○ Total Fat 18g
  Saturated Fat 10g

○ Sodium 123mg

SERVING TIP
Accompany each serving of the tart with a spoonful of plain yogurt or low fat crème fraîche.

Preparation Time: 1 hour, plus 15 minutes cooling
Serves: 12

FOR THE PASTRY
¾ cup (100g) all-purpose flour
1 tbsp cocoa powder
4 tbsp (60g) unsalted butter
¼ cup (30g) ground almonds
2 tbsp (30g) sugar
1 egg, beaten

FOR THE FILLING
3 ripe pears, peeled, cored, and cut into thick slices
4 tbsp (60g) unsalted butter
7oz (200g) semisweet chocolate, broken into pieces
3 eggs, separated
3 tbsp (45g) sugar
6 tbsp low fat crème fraîche
1 tsp ground cinnamon
powdered sugar, to dust

1 Preheat the oven to 400°F/200°C. Lightly grease the base and sides of a 1in (2.5cm) deep 9in (23cm) fluted tart pan.

2 Put all the dry ingredients for the pastry in a mixing bowl, add the lightly beaten egg, and mix everything together to form a firm dough. Alternatively, mix together all the ingredients for the pastry in a food processor until a ball of dough is formed. Turn the dough out on to a lightly floured surface and knead briefly. Roll out the dough into a circle large enough to fit the prepared tart pan.

3 Roll up the dough around a rolling pin, lay it over the tart pan, and press it into the base and sides. Bake the pastry shell blind for 10 minutes. Remove from the oven and place on a wire rack.

4 Arrange the pear slices over the bottom of the pastry shell.

5 Put the butter and chocolate in a ovenproof bowl set over a pan of simmering water. While the butter and chocolate are melting, whisk the egg whites until stiff.

6 Beat together the egg yolks, sugar, crème fraîche, and cinnamon, then beat in the melted chocolate mixture. Fold in the egg whites. Pour the mixture over the pears in the pastry shell.

7 Return the tart pan to the oven and bake for 20 minutes. The tart filling will look a little runny at this stage, but will set as it cools. Cool the tart on a wire rack before serving it dusted with powdered sugar.

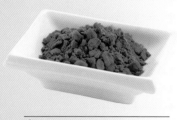

CHOCOLATE CREPES WITH APPLE & APRICOT FILLING

EACH SERVING PROVIDES:

○ Calories 209

○ Protein 8g

○ Carbohydrate 37g
  Fiber 2g

○ Total Fat 4g
  Saturated Fat 2g

○ Sodium 110mg

PREPARATION TIP

The cooked pancakes may be frozen for 3 months.

Preparation Time: 40 minutes, plus 30 minutes chilling
Serves: 5

FOR THE BATTER
1 cup (125g) all-purpose flour
2 tbsp cocoa powder
1 egg
1 egg yolk
1¼ cups (300ml) skim milk
1 tbsp olive oil, plus a little extra for cooking

FOR THE FILLING
2 cooking apples, peeled, cored, and coarsely chopped
2 tbsp sugar
½ tsp nutmeg
grated peel and juice of 1 orange
3–4 fresh apricots, pits removed and cut into quarters
powdered sugar, to dust

1 For the batter, sift the flour and cocoa powder into a large bowl and make a well in the centre. Whisk together the remaining ingredients. Pour the mixture into the flour, and whisk until smooth. Chill for 30 minutes.

2 Meanwhile, make the filling. Put the apples in a heavy saucepan with the sugar, nutmeg, and grated orange peel and juice. Bring the mixture to a boil, reduce the heat, cover, and simmer for 3 minutes. Add the apricots and continue cooking for 3 minutes, until the fruit is tender.

3 Brush a non-stick frying pan with a little oil and heat it. Pour in a little of the batter and tip the pan so that the batter covers the base. Cook over a medium heat for 1–2 minutes, until the mixture has started to bubble, then flip the crêpe over with a spatula and cook the other side. Tip the cooked crêpe onto waxed paper and make more crêpes in the same way. The mixture should make 10 crêpes.

4 Serve the pancakes filled with the apple and apricot mixture and dusted lightly with the powdered sugar.

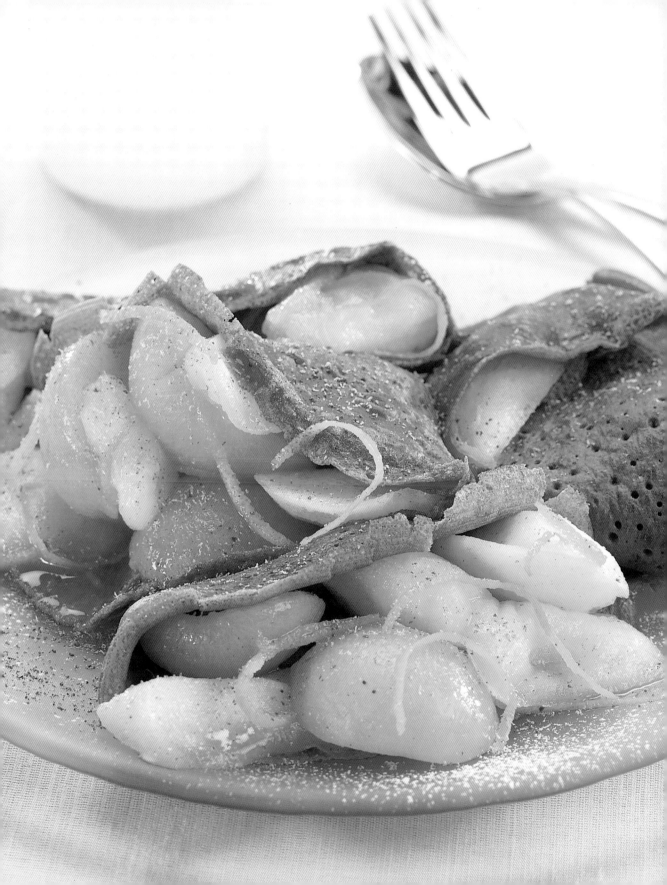

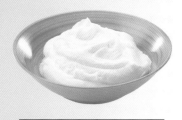

TROPICAL FRUIT & AMARETTI TRIFLE

THIS CONTEMPORARY VARIATION ON THE CLASSIC ENGLISH TRIFLE

IS SUITABLE BOTH FOR FESTIVE OCCASIONS AND FOR

EASY ENTERTAINING.

*15oz (475g) can pineapple chunks
in natural juice*
2 kiwis, peeled and chopped
1 mango, peeled and chopped
*1 piece preserved ginger in syrup, finely
chopped, and 2 tbsp of the syrup*
7oz (200g) amaretti cookies, crushed
8oz (250g) mascarpone
1lb (500g) plain yogurt
2 tbsp powdered sugar
*$^{1}/_{4}$ cup (30g) flaked almonds, toasted,
to decorate*

1 Drain the pineapple, reserving 3 tablespoons of the juice. Put the pineapple in a serving bowl with the other fruit, reserved juice, stem ginger, and ginger syrup. Combine well.

2 Scatter the crushed amaretti biscuits over the fruits.

3 Beat together the mascarpone, yogurt, and powdered sugar. Spoon the mixture over the crushed cookies and fruit, spreading it smoothly. Chill in the refrigerator for 30 minutes.

4 Before serving, decorate the trifle with the toasted almonds.

✳ STAR INGREDIENT
Plain yogurt is a good substitute for cream, the traditional trifle topping. It is lower in fat and also higher in protein and calcium.

EACH SERVING PROVIDES:

○ Calories 287

○ Protein 8g

○ Carbohydrate 25g
　Fiber 2g

○ Total Fat 18g
　Saturated Fat 8g

○ Sodium 129mg

PREPARATION TIP
This dessert may be made the day before it is required and kept in the refrigerator.

Preparation Time: 20 minutes, plus 30 minutes chilling
Serves: 8

TASTY TIRAMISU

EACH SERVING PROVIDES:

○ Calories 177

○ Protein 9g

○ Carbohydrate 17g
 Fiber 0g

○ Total Fat 8g
 Saturated Fat 5g

○ Sodium 28mg

SERVING TIP
Make the Tiramisu in one
large serving dish, if desired.
For a dessert serving 8–10,
double the recipe quantities.

Preparation Time: 15 minutes,
plus 5 minutes soaking
Serves: 4

6 ladyfingers, halved
6 tbsp strong black coffee
2 tbsp marsala
1 cup (200g) virtually fat-free fromage frais
1 cup (200g) low fat cream cheese
2 tbsp sugar
2 tbsp cocoa powder
2 tbsp grated semisweet chocolate

1 Divide the ladyfingers among 4 individual serving dishes.

2 Mix together the coffee and 1 tablespoon of the marsala and pour over the cookies. Set aside to soak for 5 minutes.

3 Meanwhile, beat together the fromage frais, cream cheese, sugar, and remaining marsala. Spoon a little of the mixture over the lady-fingers, then sieve over a little cocoa powder.

4 Continue to layer the cheese mixture and the cocoa powder, finishing with a layer of cocoa powder. Scatter the grated chocolate over the top. Chill before serving.

SPICED FRUIT KEBABS

EACH SERVING PROVIDES:

○ Calories 95

○ Protein 1g

○ Carbohydrate 23g
 Fiber 3g

○ Total Fat 0g
 Saturated Fat 0g

○ Sodium 6mg

SERVING TIP
This dessert is delicious served
with a little vanilla ice cream
or a spoonful of Greek yogurt.

Preparation Time: 20 minutes
Serves: 4

3 fresh figs, quartered
1 small pineapple, peeled, cored, and cut into chunks
2 pears, peeled, cored, and cut into chunks
8 large strawberries
grated peel and juice of 1 orange
1 tsp ground cinnamon
2 tbsp honey

1 Thread the fruits alternately on to 8 wooden skewers. Mix together the grated orange peel and juice, cinnamon, and honey and drizzle over the fruit kebabs.

2 Place the kebabs under a preheated broiler and broil for 5–6 minutes, turning them occasionally and brushing frequently with the honey mixture, until they begin to brown. Serve at once.

PANNA COTTA

EACH SERVING PROVIDES:

○ Calories 275

○ Protein 4g

○ Carbohydrate 16g
   Fiber 0g

○ Total Fat 20g
   Saturated Fat 12g

○ Sodium 137mg

Preparation Time: 15 minutes, plus 15 minutes cooling and 1–2 hours chilling
Serves: 6

Illustrated right

8oz (250g) mascarpone
1/3 cup (75g) sugar
1 tsp vanilla extract
1 cup (200g) virtually fat-free fromage frais
grated peel and juice of 1 orange
1/2 envelope (3.5g) gelatine
fresh berry fruits, to serve

1 Put the mascarpone, sugar, and vanilla extract in a heavy-based saucepan and heat gently until the sugar has dissolved. Remove from the heat and set aside to cool for 15 minutes.

2 Whisk in the fromage frais.

3 Place the grated orange peel and juice in a small bowl and sprinkle the gelatine on top. Leave for 2–3 minutes until spongy, then place over a pan of simmering water until the gelatine has dissolved.

4 Quickly whisk the gelatine mixture into the mascarpone mixture. Pour into 6 individual-size ramekins or molds and chill for 1–2 hours to set.

5 Dip the molds in hot water for a few seconds and turn the panna cottas out on to dessert plates. Serve with the berry fruits.

BANANA & LEMON BRULEE

EACH SERVING PROVIDES:

○ Calories 119

○ Protein 1g

○ Carbohydrate 18g
   Fiber 0g

○ Total Fat 5g
   Saturated Fat 3g

○ Sodium 17mg

PREPARATION TIP
To make Banana and Orange Brulée, replace the lemon curd with orange curd and the lemon peel with orange peel.

Preparation Time: 15 minutes, plus 30 minutes chilling
Serves: 4

1 large banana, sliced
1 cup (200g) low fat crème fraîche
2 tbsp lemon curd
grated peel of 1 lemon
4 tsp brown sugar

1 Divide the banana slices among 4 heatproof ramekin dishes.

2 Beat together the crème fraîche, lemon curd, and grated lemon peel. Spoon the mixture over the banana slices. Chill for 30 minutes.

3 Sprinkle the sugar over the crème fraîche mixture. Put the ramekins under a preheated broiler and broil for 1–2 minutes, until the sugar has caramelized. Return the ramekins to the refrigerator for the caramel to cool and set, then serve.

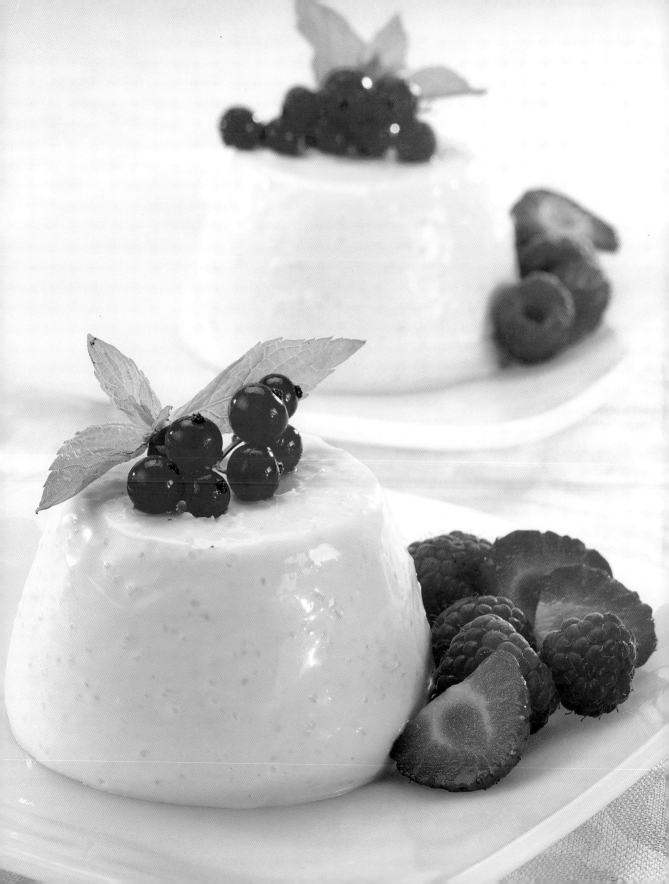

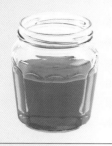

BAKED PEACH PACKETS

THIS EYE-CATCHING WAY OF SERVING INDIVIDUAL HOT FRUIT DESSERTS

IS GOOD FOR INFORMAL ENTERTAINING – GUESTS WON'T

QUICKLY FORGET THE OCCASION.

4 peaches, halved and pitted
2 tbsp honey
grated peel and juice of 1 orange
2 tbsp (30g) unsalted butter
¹/₂ cup (100g) plain yogurt
1 tsp vanilla extract
about 8 (60g) amaretti cookies,
lightly crushed, to decorate

1 Preheat the oven to 400°F/200°C. Cut out 4 pieces of foil, each about 10in (26cm) square. Put 2 peach halves in the center of each piece and bring up the sides of the foil slightly.

2 Put the honey, grated orange peel and juice, and butter in a small saucepan and heat gently until the butter has melted.

3 Divide the honey mixture among the peach packets and fold the foil to enclose the peaches. Put the foil packets in a shallow baking dish. Bake for 10–12 minutes, until the peaches are tender.

4 Open up the packets and set them on individual dessert plates. Mix together the yogurt and vanilla and spoon over the peaches. Scatter the crushed amaretti cookies over the top and serve.

✷ STAR INGREDIENT
Although honey is high in sugar, it has a distinctive, rich flavor and so can be used in smaller amounts than other sugars.

EACH SERVING PROVIDES:

○ Calories 173

○ Protein 3g

○ Carbohydrate 19g
  Fiber 2g

○ Total Fat 9g
  Saturated Fat 5g

○ Sodium 80mg

PREPARATION TIP
Instead of making individual parcels, bake the peaches in a single layer in an ovenproof dish, covered with foil.

Preparation Time: 30 minutes
Serves: 4

SIMPLE CITRUS TERRINE

1 packet of lemon gelatin dessert
²/₃ cup (150ml) boiling water
grated peel and juice of 1 lime
1¹/₂ cups (400g) light evaporated milk, chilled

TO DECORATE
²/₃ cup (150ml) whipping cream,
whipped to form soft peaks
lemon slices
lime slices

1 Line a 2lb (1kg) loaf pan with plastic wrap. Dissolve the gelatin dessert mix in the boiling water and stir in the grated lime peel and juice. Let it cool.

2 Meanwhile, whisk the evaporated milk until it has doubled in volume, then gradually whisk in the cooled gelatin dessert.

3 Pour the mixture into the prepared pan and put in the refrigerator to set, about 2–3 hours. To serve, turn the terrine out on to a serving dish and decorate with the whipped cream and the lemon and lime slices.

EACH SERVING PROVIDES:

○ Calories 162

○ Protein 5g

○ Carbohydrate 15g
   Fiber 0g

○ Total Fat 8g
   Saturated Fat 4g

○ Sodium 100mg

PREPARATION TIP
Chill the evaporated milk in the refrigerator overnight to make it easier to beat and to allow the terrine to set more quickly.

Preparation Time: 20 minutes, plus 2–3 hours setting.
Serves: 8

PAPAYA & PASSION FRUIT COMPOTE WITH BASIL

¹/₄ cup (60g) sugar
²/₃ cup (150ml) water
few drops vanilla extract
2 papayas, peeled, seeded, and chopped
1 tbsp chopped fresh basil
flesh of 2 passion fruits

1 Put the sugar, water, and vanilla in a small, heavy-bottomed saucepan, bring slowly to a boil, then reduce the heat and simmer gently for 2 minutes.

2 Stir in the remaining ingredients. Serve the compote hot or cold.

EACH SERVING PROVIDES:

○ Calories 88

○ Protein 1g

○ Carbohydrate 23g
   Fiber 2g

○ Total Fat 0g
   Saturated Fat 0g

○ Sodium 6mg

PREPARATION TIPS
Use mangoes, pears, or other fruits in place of the papaya.

Preparation Time: 15 minutes
Serves: 4

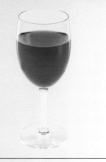

SPICED POACHED PEARS WITH VANILLA MINT CREAM

ALTHOUGH THESE SPICY PEARS HAVE A REAL FEEL OF CHRISTMAS,

THEY MAKE A FESTIVE DESSERT WHATEVER THE SEASON.

4 large, firm pears,
peeled and with the stems left on
12 cloves
1 cinnamon stick
grated peel and juice of 1 orange
1¼ cups (300ml) red wine
2 tbsp honey

FOR THE MINT CREAM
6 tbsp low fat crème fraîche
few drops vanilla extract
1 tbsp chopped fresh mint

1 Stud each pear with 3 cloves. Place in a saucepan with the cinnamon stick, grated orange peel and juice, and red wine.

2 Bring to a boil, reduce the heat, and simmer gently until the pears are tender. Let the pears cool in the liquid, then remove them from the pan.

3 With the pan uncovered, boil the cooking liquid until it has reduced by half. Stir in the honey.

4 Mix together all the ingredients for the mint cream in a small bowl.

5 Serve the pears drizzled with a little of the thickened juice and with a spoonful of mint cream.

★ STAR INGREDIENT
Alcohol such as red wine is an excellent flavor enhancer in recipes intended for special-occasions meals or for celebrations.

EACH SERVING PROVIDES:

- ○ Calories 221
- ○ Protein 2g
- ○ Carbohydrate 33g
  Fiber 5g
- ○ Total Fat 5g
  Saturated Fat 3g
- ○ Sodium 23mg

SERVING TIP
Vanilla ice cream is a delicious accompaniment for these pears, in place of the vanilla mint cream.

Preparation Time: 25 minutes,
Serves: 4

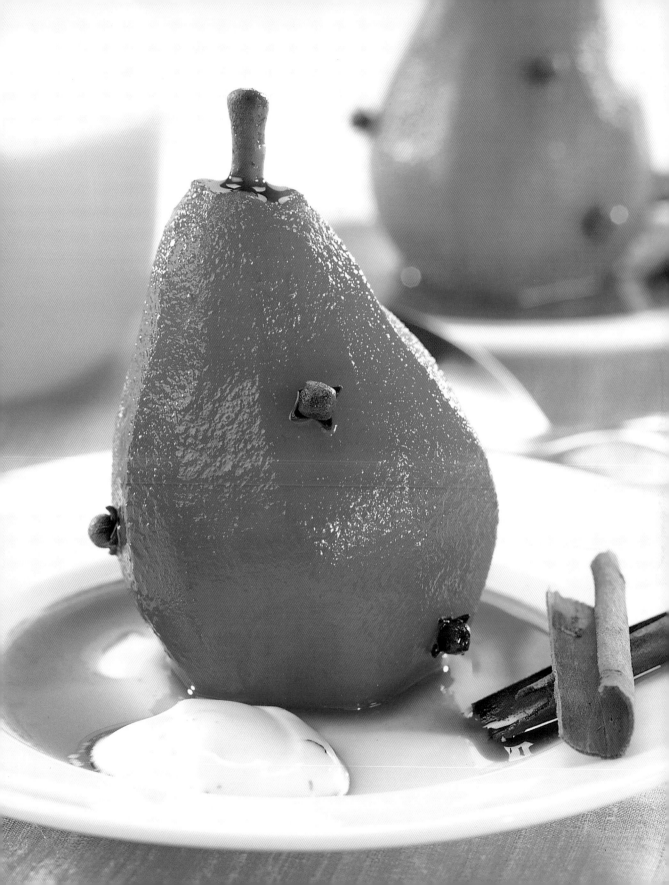

Fruit Sabayon

EACH SERVING PROVIDES:

○ Calories 173

○ Protein 3g

○ Carbohydrate 26g
   Fiber 2g

○ Total Fat 5g
   Saturated Fat 3g

○ Sodium 13mg

PREPARATION TIP
If using canned rather than fresh fruits, choose fruits in natural juice, not syrup.

Preparation Time: 20 minutes
Serves: 6

3 cups (750g) mixed fresh apricots and nectarines, stoned and sliced

3 egg yolks

⅓ cup (75g) sugar

grated peel of 1 lime

1 cup (200ml) dry white wine

⅔ cup (150ml) light cream

① Scatter the fruit over the bottom of a 1 quart (1.8 liter) shallow, ovenproof dish.

② Put the egg yolks and sugar in a heatproof bowl and set over a pan of simmering water. Whisk together lightly.

③ Add the grated lime peel and wine and whisk for about 10 minutes, keeping the water just simmering, until the mixture is light, airy, and thick enough for the whisk to leave a trail on the surface.

④ Remove from the heat and whisk in the cream.

⑤ Pour the egg mixture over the fruit in the ovenproof dish and put under a preheated broiler. Broil for 2–3 minutes, until the top is dark golden. Serve the sabayon immediately.

Plum Crumble

EACH SERVING PROVIDES:

○ Calories 278

○ Protein 4g

○ Carbohydrate 43g
   Fiber 3g

○ Total Fat 11g
   Saturated Fat 7g

○ Sodium 100mg

PREPARATION TIP
For a more crunchy topping, replace the rolled oats with the same quantity of muesli.

Preparation Time: 40–45 minutes
Serves: 6

1lb (500g) fresh plums, quartered and pitted
¾ cup (100g) all-purpose flour
5 tbsp (75g) unsalted butter
½ cup (75g) light brown sugar
⅓ cup (75g) rolled oats
1 tsp ground cinnamon

① Preheat the oven to 400°F/200°C. Arrange the plums in an ovenproof dish.

② Rub together the flour and butter with your fingertips, until the mixture resembles fine breadcrumbs. Add the sugar, oats, and cinnamon and stir well together. Scatter the mixture over the plums, pressing it down lightly.

③ Bake for 30–35 minutes, or until the top is golden. Serve the crumble with a little ice cream or yogurt, if desired.

APRICOT PUDDING

THIS FRUITY STEAMED PUDDING IS QUICK TO MAKE, EASY

TO COOK, AND VERY DELICIOUS – WHAT MORE NEEDS TO

BE ASKED OF A DESSERT?

1 cup (250g) dried apricots, chopped
grated peel and juice of 1 orange
3 tbsp water
7 tbsp (100g) margarine
½ cup (75g) light brown sugar
2 eggs, beaten
1½ cups (180g) self-rising flour
1 tsp cinnamon
2 tbsp corn syrup

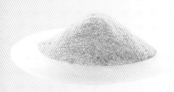

★ STAR INGREDIENT
There is no need to replace sugar, whatever the kind, with alternative sweeteners in baking. Most recipes work well with reduced amounts of sugar (see page 24).

EACH SERVING PROVIDES:

○ Calories 394

○ Protein 7g

○ Carbohydrate 58g
  Fiber 4g

○ Total Fat 16g
  Saturated Fat 4g

○ Sodium 177mg

PREPARATION TIP
To shorten the cooking time, steam the pudding in a microwave oven. Cook it, uncovered, on High for 7–8 minutes, and let stand for 5 minutes before serving.

Preparation Time: 2 hours
Serves: 6

1 Put the apricots in a small saucepan with the grated orange peel and juice and the water. Bring to a boil, turn down the heat, and simmer gently for 5 minutes, until the liquid has been absorbed.

2 For the sponge, beat together the margarine, sugar, eggs, flour, and cinnamon until the mixture is light and fluffy.

3 Stir the corn syrup into the apricots, then put in a lightly greased, 6 cup (1.5 litre) pudding mold. Spoon the sponge mixture over the apricots and smooth the top. Put a double-thickness layer of waxed paper, with a pleat across the middle, over the pudding mold and tie tightly with string.

4 Lower the pudding into a saucepan filled with enough boiling water to come halfway up the side of the pudding mold; alternatively, put the mold in the top half of a steamer. Cover the pan and steam the pudding for 1½ hours, adding more boiling water, if necessary, during cooking.

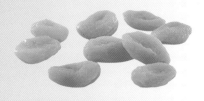

BAKED ST. CLEMENT'S CHEESECAKE

THIS IS A REDUCED-FAT VERSION OF A FAVORITE FAMILY CHEESECAKE.

DECORATE IT EXTRAVAGANTLY AND IT BECOMES

A SPLENDID CELEBRATION DESSERT.

4tbsp (60g) unsalted butter
10 (180g) ginger cookies, crushed
2 x 8oz (250g) cartons Quark (virtually fat-free soft cheese);
or use 1lb (500g) low fat cottage cheese, puréed)
4oz (125g) sugar
2 eggs
grated peel and juice of 2 oranges
grated peel and juice of 2 lemons
$^1/_2$ cup (100g) ready-to-eat dried apricots, chopped

To Decorate
slices of orange and lemon, lightly poached
strips of orange and lemon peel, lightly poached
a little powdered sugar, to dust

1 Preheat the oven to 300°F/150°C. Lightly grease an 8in (20cm) non-stick, springform tart pan.

2 Melt the butter in a small saucepan, stir in the cookie crumbs, and mix well together. Press the mixture into the bottom and about halfway up the sides of the tart pan. Bake for 10 minutes.

3 Beat together the cheese, caster sugar, eggs, and grated orange and lemon peels and juices until smooth. Stir in the chopped apricots.

4 Spoon the mixture on to the cookie crust in the tart pan, return the pan to the oven, and bake for 40 minutes. Turn off the oven and leave the cheesecake in it for 1 hour to cool.

5 Chill the cheesecake in the refrigerator for 2 hours before serving. Arrange the orange and lemon slices and strips of peel decoratively on top, then dust with the powdered sugar.

✳ STAR INGREDIENT
Dried fruits like apricots are high in fiber and antioxidants such as beta-carotene.

EACH SERVING PROVIDES:

○ Calories 246

○ Protein 10g

○ Carbohydrate 33g
  Fibre 1g

○ Total Fat 9g
  Saturated Fat 5g

○ Sodium 146mg

SERVING TIP
For citrus decorations with a difference, sprinkle a little sugar over the citrus slices and peel for the top of the cheesecake and broil them for a few minutes until the sugar is lightly browned.

Preparation Time: 1¼ hours, plus 1 hour cooling and 2 hours chilling
Serves: 10

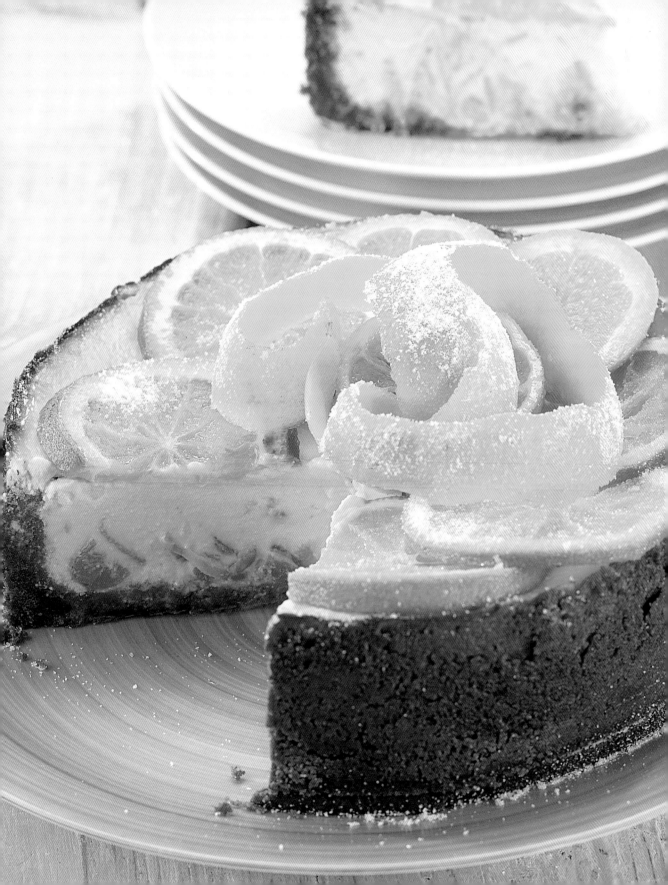

∗ STAR INGREDIENT
Sun-dried tomatoes, like dried fruit, are a good source of antioxidant vitamins, except vitamin C. Those in oil can be used at once; those sold dried loose need 20–30 minutes' soaking before use.

EACH WEDGE PROVIDES:

- Calories 242
- Protein 7g
- Carbohydrate 47g
  Fiber 2g
- Total Fat 2g
  Saturated Fat 0.5g
- Sodium 44mg

SERVING TIP
This bread is delicious eaten warm. Serve it with one of the soups in the chapter on appetizers for a satisfying light meal or snack.

Preparation Time: 55 minutes plus 1 hour first rise and 20 minutes second rise
Makes: 2 loaves (each loaf gives 6 wedges)

SUN-DRIED TOMATO & ROSEMARY BREAD

6 cups (750g) bread flour
pinch of salt
pinch of sugar
1/2 tbsp chopped fresh rosemary
8 sun-dried tomatoes in oil,
drained and chopped

1 package (7g) dried yeast
1 tbsp olive oil
2 cups (450ml) warm water
milk, for brushing

1 Sift together the flour, salt, and sugar in a large bowl. Stir in the rosemary, sun-dried tomatoes, and yeast. Make a well in the center of the mixture. Mix the oil with the warm water and pour into the well in the flour mixture. Quickly mix in the flour to form a soft dough.

2 Turn the dough onto a lightly floured surface and knead for about 6 minutes, until the dough is smooth and elastic. Put the dough in a lightly oiled bowl, cover with a damp cloth, and set aside to rise for about 1 hour, until doubled in size.

3 Preheat the oven to 425°F/220°C. Reknead the dough for 3 minutes, then divide it into 2 pieces. Shape each piece of dough into a large oval shape and cut 2 slashes on the top of each to make an "X". Place the loaves on a lightly floured baking sheet, cover, and let rise for about 20 minutes, until doubled in size.

4 Brush the risen loaves with a little milk. Bake in the oven for 35 minutes, or until the loaves sound hollow when tapped underneath. Leave the loaves on a wire rack to cool slightly.

BAKING
Most baking includes some sugar or high-fat ingredients, which you should limit in your diet if you are overweight. These recipes show how you can reduce such ingredients and increase fiber content while retaining all the delicious flavors of home baking.

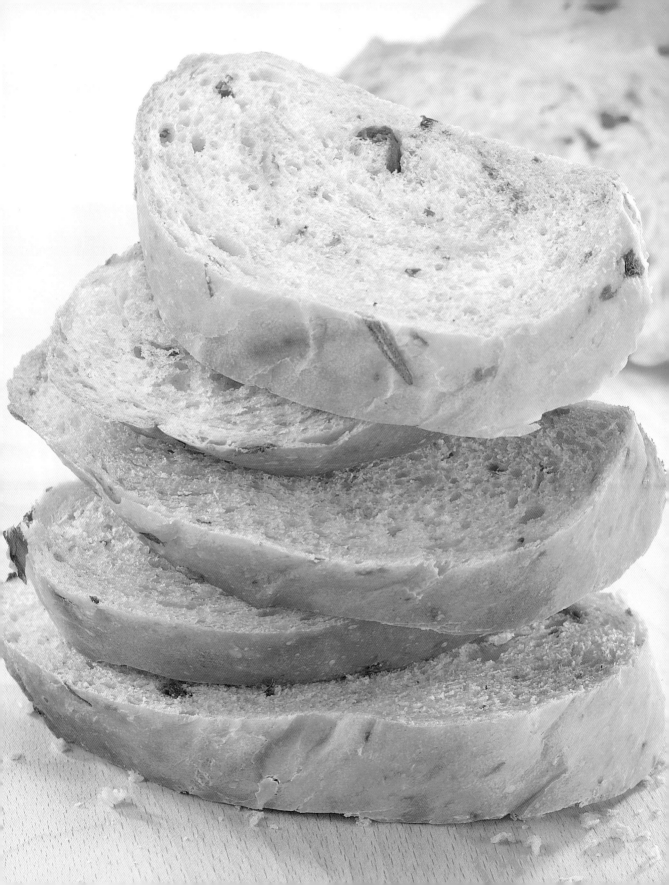

WALNUT BREAD

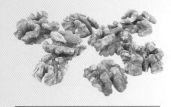

2²/₃ cups (300g) whole wheat flour
2¹/₂ cups (300g) all-purpose flour
1 tsp salt
1 package (7g) dried yeast
1 tbsp brown sugar
1¹/₂ cups (180g) walnut pieces
1 tbsp walnut oil
1³/₄ cups (400ml) lukewarm water

★ STAR INGREDIENT
Walnuts contain omega-3 polyunsaturated fatty acids (*see pages 18–19*), which are believed to reduce the risk of heart attacks and blood clots.

EACH SLICE PROVIDES:

○ Calories 211

○ Protein 6g

○ Carbohydrate 28g
  Fiber 3g

○ Total Fat 9g
  Saturated Fat 1g

○ Sodium 2mg

PREPARATION TIP
This recipe quantity will make 2 smaller loaves. Half-fill the loaf pan for a smaller loaf, and use the remaining dough to make a free-form loaf. The baking time will be about 10 minutes less than for the larger loaf.

Preparation Time: 1 hour 5 minutes–1 hour 10 minutes, plus 1¹/₂ hours first rise and 45 minutes second rise.
Makes: 1 x 2lb (1kg) loaf (16 slices)

① Lightly grease a 2lb (1kg) loaf pan and line it with waxed paper.

② Sift the flours and salt in a large bowl. Stir in the yeast, sugar, and walnut pieces. Make a well in the center of the mixture. Mix the oil with the water, pour into the well in the flour, and bring all the ingredients together to form a soft ball of dough (*see step 1, below*).

③ Turn the dough onto a floured surface and knead for 5 minutes, until smooth (*see step 2, below*). Place the dough in a lightly oiled bowl, cover, and leave for 1¹/₂–2 hours in a warm place, until doubled in size.

④ Reknead the dough for 3 minutes, shape it into a rectangle, and put in the prepared loaf pan. Let it rise for about 45 minutes, until doubled in size. Meanwhile, preheat the oven to 400°F/200°C.

⑤ Bake the bread for 45–50 minutes. Remove from the pan and return to the oven for 5 minutes. When baked, the loaf should sound hollow when tapped underneath. Cool the loaf on a wire rack.

MIXING & KNEADING BREAD DOUGH

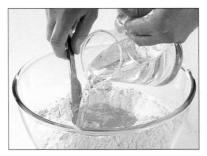

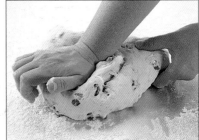

1 Use a flat-bladed knife to mix the oil and water into the dry ingredients for the bread. Employ a cutting and turning movement to form a soft ball of dough.

2 To knead the dough, use the heel of one hand to push the dough gently away from you. At the same time, use the other hand to rotate the dough around in a circle.

SUNFLOWER SEED, CHEESE & HERB LOAF

EACH SLICE PROVIDES:

○ Calories 125

○ Protein 5g

○ Carbohydrate 10g
Fiber 1g

○ Total Fat 8g
Saturated Fat 2g

○ Sodium 81mg

PREPARATION TIP
This bread is best made with a strong-flavored cheese. Alternatives to Cheddar are hard cheeses such as double Gloucester and Parmesan.

Preparation Time: 55–65 minutes
Makes: 1 x 1kg (2lb) loaf (16 slices)

THIS EASY-TO-MAKE BREAD IS A DELICIOUS ALTERNATIVE TO BREAD AND CHEESE. IT MAKES A GOOD ACCOMPANIMENT TO APPETIZERS AND MAIN DISHES THAT DO NOT INCLUDE CARBOHYDRATE.

$^{3}/_{4}$ cup (100g) all-purpose flour
$^{2}/_{3}$ cup (100g) whole wheat flour
1 tsp bicarbonate of soda
$^{1}/_{2}$ tsp cream of tartar
$^{1}/_{2}$ tsp dry mustard
4 tbsp (60g) margarine
4 tbsp chopped fresh parsley
1 cup (100g) sharp cheddar cheese, grated
5 scallions, sliced
$^{1}/_{2}$ cup (60g) sunflower seeds, toasted
1 egg, beaten
$^{2}/_{3}$ cup (150ml) 1% or skim milk

1 Preheat the oven to 400°F/200°C. Lightly grease a 2lb (1kg) loaf pan.

2 In a large bowl, sift together the flours, bicarbonate of soda, cream of tartar, and dry mustard. Rub in the margarine with your fingertips until the mixture resembles fine breadcrumbs. Stir in the parsley, cheese, scallions, and sunflower seeds.

3 Whisk together the egg and milk and pour into the bowl. Mix in the dry ingredients thoroughly to form a soft dough.

4 Transfer the dough to the prepared loaf pan. Bake for 35–40 minutes, or until a skewer comes out clean when inserted into the middle of the loaf.

5 Leave the loaf in the pan for a few minutes, then turn out onto a wire rack to cool slightly. The bread is delicious eaten warm.

CORNMEAL BRAIDS

EACH SERVING PROVIDES:

○ Calories 322

○ Protein 9g

○ Carbohydrate 61g
  Fiber 2g

○ Total Fat 6g
  Saturated Fat 3g

○ Sodium 57mg

SERVING TIP
This cornmeal bread is best served fresh. Eat it the day it is made, or freeze it and use within 3 months.

Preparation Time: 55 minutes, plus 1½ hours rising
Makes: 2 braids; each serves 6

2¼ cups (375g) cornmeal
4 cups (500g) bread flour
¼ cup (60g) light brown sugar
2 packages (15g) dried yeast

pinch of salt
4 tbsp (60g) butter, cut into cubes
1⅔ cups (375ml) warm
1% or skim milk

1 Place all but 1 tablespoon of the cornmeal in a large bowl with the flour, sugar, yeast, and salt. Mix together well. Rub in the butter with your fingertips until the mixture resembles fine breadcrumbs. Add the milk and stir the ingredients together to form a soft dough.

2 Turn the dough out onto a lightly floured surface and knead for 5 minutes, until smooth.

3 Divide the dough into 6 pieces and roll each out to a rope about 12in (30cm) long. Lay 3 of the ropes of dough on a lightly floured surface and braid them (*see steps 1 and 2, below*). Make a second braid with the remaining 3 dough ropes.

4 Place the loaves on a lightly floured baking sheet, cover with a damp cloth, and leave in a warm place for 1½ hours, until doubled in size. Meanwhile, preheat the oven to 450°F/230°C.

5 Brush each loaf with water, then sprinkle over the reserved cornmeal. Bake for 15 minutes. Reduce the oven temperature to 375°F/190°C and bake for a further 15 minutes. Cool the loaves on a wire rack.

MAKING THE DOUGH PLAITS

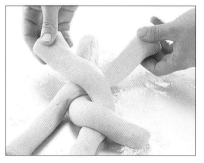

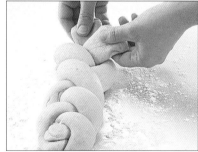

1 To braid the dough, start from the center of the ropes and twist them into braids down to one end. Turn the dough around and braid along to the other end.

2 At each end of the completed loaf, turn the ends of the dough under to form neat ends.

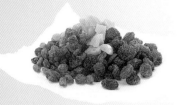

Fruity Tea Bread

LOW IN FAT YET DELICIOUSLY MOIST, THIS TEA BREAD IS AN IDEAL

FAMILY TREAT. SERVE IT WITH TEA OR COFFEE, OR WITH A GLASS

OF MILK AS AN AFTER-SCHOOL SNACK FOR CHILDREN.

12 tbsp cold strong tea

1lb (500g) mixed dried fruits,
such as raisins, chopped apricots,
and golden raisins

$^2/_3$ cup (150g) sugar

1 egg, beaten

2 tbsp (30g) unsalted butter, melted

2 cups (250g) all-purpose flour

1 tsp bicarbonate of soda

1 Put the tea, fruit, and sugar in a large bowl and mix together well. Cover and set aside overnight for the fruits to soak in the tea.

2 The next day, lightly grease a 2lb (1kg) loaf pan and line it with waxed paper. Preheat the oven to 350°F/180°C.

3 Add all the remaining ingredients to the bowl of soaked fruit and stir them in well. Spoon the mixture into the prepared loaf pan. Bake for 1½ hours, or until a skewer inserted into the center of the loaf comes out clean.

4 Cool the loaf for 10 minutes in the pan, then transfer it to a wire rack to finish cooling.

✸ STAR INGREDIENT
Dried mixed fruits are good sources of fiber, vitamins, and minerals such as iron.

EACH SLICE PROVIDES:

○ Calories 177

○ Protein 3g

○ Carbohydrate 39g
  Fiber 2g

○ Total Fat 2g
  Saturated Fat 1g

○ Sodium 32mg

SERVING TIP
There is no need to eat this bread with extra butter, since the dried fruit makes it moist.

Preparation Time: 1¾ hours, plus overnight soaking
Makes: 1 x 2lb (1kg) loaf (16 slices)

BANANA, OAT & HONEY MUFFINS

2 cups (250g) all-purpose flour

⅓ cup (75g) rolled oats

1 tbsp baking powder

½ tsp grated nutmeg

2 medium bananas, mashed

1 egg, beaten

5 tbsp (75g) unsalted butter, melted

1oz (30g) dark brown sugar

¾ cup (175ml) buttermilk

3 tbsp honey

1 Preheat the oven to 400°F/200°C. Lightly grease and flour a tray of 12 muffin pans.

2 Put the flour, oats, baking powder, and nutmeg in a large bowl and mix together well.

3 Mix together all the remaining ingredients. Use a spoon to fold them through the flour mixture, until just combined.

4 Spoon the mixture into the prepared muffin pans. Bake for about 20 minutes, until the muffins have risen and are golden. Cool in the muffin pans for 10 minutes before serving.

WHITE CHOCOLATE & PECAN NUT MINI-MUFFINS

2 cups (250g) all-purpose flour

2 tsp baking powder

½ tsp baking soda

5oz (150g) white chocolate, roughly chopped

1 cup (100g) pecan nuts, chopped

1 tsp vanilla extract

2 eggs, beaten

⅓ cup (275ml) buttermilk

¼ cup (60g) light brown sugar

5 tbsp (75g) unsalted butter, melted

1 Preheat the oven to 400°F/200°C. Lightly grease and flour 3 trays of 12 mini-muffin pans. (If you have only 1 pan, bake the muffins in batches; the mixture can be left unbaked for this amount of time.)

2 Sift together the flour, baking powder, and baking soda in a large bowl. Stir in the chocolate and nuts. Whisk together the remaining ingredients and quickly fold them into the flour mixture.

3 Spoon the mixture into the prepared mini-muffin pans. Bake for 12–15 minutes, until golden and risen. Cool the muffins in the pans on a wire rack for 10 minutes then serve.

EACH MUFFIN PROVIDES:

○ Calories 190

○ Protein 4g

○ Carbohydrate 31g
   Fiber 1g

○ Total Fat 7g
   Saturated Fat 4g

○ Sodium 66mg

PREPARATION TIP

If preferred, spoon the mixture into paper muffin cases and put the cases on an ungreased muffin tray for baking.

Preparation Time: 30 minutes
Makes: 12

Illustrated right

EACH MUFFIN PROVIDES:

○ Calories 87

○ Protein 2g

○ Carbohydrate 10g
   Fiber 0g

○ Total Fat 5g
   Saturated Fat 2g

○ Sodium 28mg

PREPARATION TIP

Replace the white chocolate with plain chocolate for a change of flavor.

Preparation Time: 30–35 minutes
Makes: 36

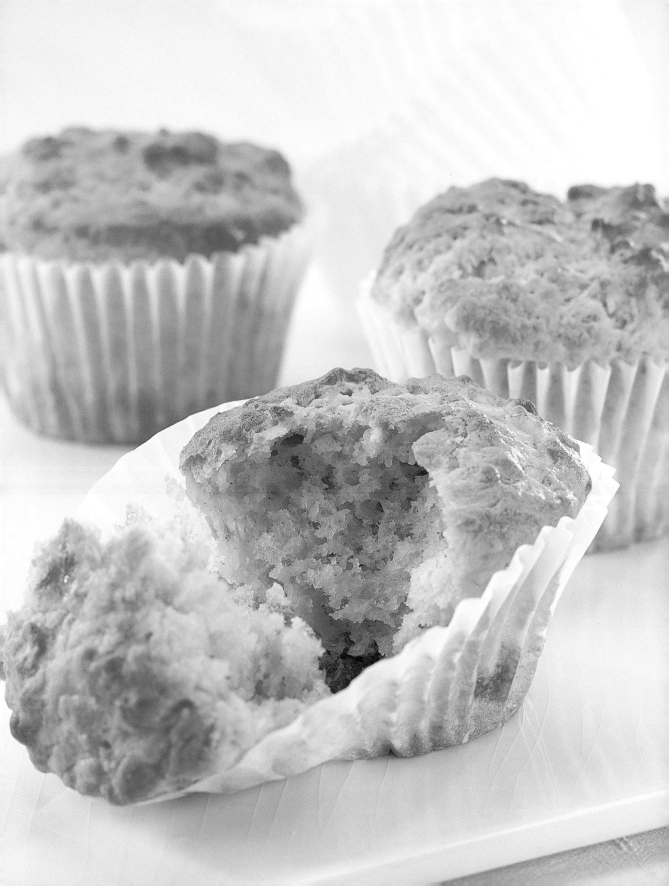

CHERRY & COCONUT CAKE

THIS IS A GOOD CAKE FOR SPECIAL DAYS, SUCH AS BIRTHDAYS.

IT FREEZES WELL, AND CAN THEREFORE BE MADE SEVERAL WEEKS

IN ADVANCE OF THE OCCASION.

*²/₃ cup (150g) glacé cherries, rinsed,
dried, and roughly chopped
2 cups (250g) self-raising flour
1 tsp baking powder
³/₄ cup (75g) grated coconut
7 tbsp (100g) margarine or unsalted butter
¹/₃ cup (75g) sugar
3 eggs, beaten
grated peel and juice of 1 lemon
a few drops vanilla extract
4 tbsp 1% or skim milk*

1 Preheat the oven to 350°F/180°C. Lightly grease and flour a deep, 7in (18cm) cake pan.

2 Mix together the cherries, the flour, the baking powder, and all but 1 tablespoon of the coconut.

3 Beat together the margarine and sugar until light and fluffy. Gradually add the eggs, beating well, and adding a little flour to the mixture if it begins to curdle.

4 Mix in the grated lemon peel and juice, vanilla extract, and milk. Fold in the flour mixture.

5 Spoon the mixture into the prepared cake pan and level the top. Scatter the reserved coconut over the top.

6 Bake in the oven for 50–60 minutes, or until a skewer inserted into the center of the cake comes out clean.

7 Cool the cake in the tin for 10 minutes. Take it out of the pan and sit it on a wire rack to complete cooling.

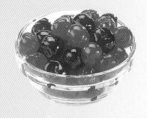

✳ STAR INGREDIENT
Glacé cherries are preserved in syrup, which is high in sugar. Rinse the cherries to remove some of the sugar so they can safely be used for people with diabetes, without harming blood glucose levels.

EACH SERVING PROVIDES:

○ Calories 290

○ Protein 5g

○ Carbohydrate 37g
   Fiber 2g

○ Total Fat 15g
   Saturated Fat 6g

○ Sodium 190mg

SERVING TIP
Store this cake in an airtight container and eat within 3 days. It also freezes well.

Preparation Time: 1 hour 5 minutes–1¹/₄ hours
Serves: 10

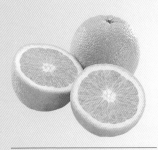

Oranges, like other citrus
fruits, are rich in vitamin C,
a vitamin that is needed
every day to help the body
to resist infection.

EACH SERVING PROVIDES:

○ Calories 240

○ Protein 4g

○ Carbohydrate 18g
　Fiber 1g

○ Total Fat 17g
　Saturated Fat 3g

○ Sodium 170mg

PREPARATION TIP
For a different flavor, replace
the grated orange peel and
juice with those of lemons or
limes. Both these citrus fruits
combine well with almonds.

Preparation Time: 1 hour
5 minutes–1¼ hours
Serves: 12

ALMOND & ORANGE CAKE

THIS REFRESHINGLY FLAVORED, MOIST CAKE SERVED WITH LOW FAT
CREME FRAICHE MAKES A DELICIOUS SPECIAL OCCASION DESSERT.

FOR THE CAKE
¾ cup (180g) margarine
⅓ cup (75g) sugar
3 eggs, beaten
1¼ cups (150g) self-rising flour
1 tsp baking powder
⅓ cup (75g) ground almonds
grated peel and juice of 1 orange
few drops almond extract

FOR THE TOPPING
grated peel and juice of 2 oranges
2 tbsp (30g) granulated sugar

1 Preheat the oven to 325°F/160°C. Lightly grease and flour a deep,
8in (20cm)) cake pan.

2 Put all the ingredients for the cake in a large bowl and beat together
thoroughly. Alternatively, put the cake ingredients in a food processor
and process until combined.

3 Spoon the mixture into the prepared cake pan. Bake for 50–60
minutes, until golden and firm to the touch.

4 Mix together the topping ingredients and drizzle over the still-warm
cake. Cool on a wire rack.

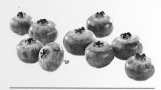

BLUEBERRY & PEAR CAKE

THIS CAKE CONTAINS FRESH FRUIT, AN IDEAL INGREDIENT IN BAKING,

PROVIDING FLAVOR, TEXTURE, AND FIBER.

1¼ cups (150g) self-rising flour
2 tsp baking powder
5 tbsp (75g) margarine
½ cup (60g) ground almonds
2 eggs
grated peel and juice of 1 orange
few drops almond extract
2 pears, peeled, cored, and chopped
1 cup (125g) blueberries
1 tbsp light brown sugar

1 Preheat the oven to 400°F/200°C. Lightly grease a deep, 8in (20cm) cake pan and line it with waxed paper.

2 Put the flour, baking powder, margarine, almonds, eggs, grated orange peel and juice, and almond extract in a large bowl and beat them together thoroughly.

3 Fold the pears and blueberries into the mixture. Spoon it into the prepared cake pan and sprinkle with the light brown sugar. Bake for 45–60 minutes, or until firm to the touch.

4 Cool the cake in the pan on a wire rack. Stored in an airtight container, it will keep for up to a week.

✳ STAR INGREDIENT
Blueberries contain a full range of B vitamins.

EACH SERVING PROVIDES:

○ Calories 181

○ Protein 4g

○ Carbohydrate 17g
Fiber 2g

○ Total Fat 11g
Saturated Fat 2g

○ Sodium 124mg

PREPARATION TIP
Replace the blueberries in this recipe with raspberries or blackberries, if desired.

Preparation Time: 1 hour 5 minutes–1 hour 20 minutes
Serves: 10

CARROT CAKE

THIS SUBSTANTIAL FAMILY FAVORITE HAS A MELLOW, MOIST TEXTURE.

QUICK AND EASY TO PREPARE, IT IS EQUALLY GOOD AS A COFFEE-TIME

SNACK, FOR CHILDREN'S PARTIES, AND IN LUNCH BOXES.

★ STAR INGREDIENT
Cottage cheese has a creamy texture and flavor, and it is available in no fat, low fat, and full fat versions.

EACH SERVING PROVIDES:

○ Calories 300

○ Protein 9g

○ Carbohydrate 20g
  Fiber 2g

○ Total Fat 20g
  Saturated Fat 4g

○ Sodium 107mg

SERVING TIP
Store this cake in an airtight container and eat within 3 days. It can be frozen for up to 3 months.

Preparation Time: 1 hour 50 minutes
Serves: 12

FOR THE CAKE
1 cup (250g) cottage cheese
$\frac{1}{2}$ cup (100g) light brown sugar
3 eggs, beaten
$1\frac{2}{3}$ cups (250g) carrots, grated
$\frac{1}{2}$ cup (100g) dried apricots, chopped
$\frac{1}{2}$ cup (75g) walnut pieces
$1\frac{1}{3}$ cups (150g) self-rising whole wheat flour
$\frac{3}{4}$ cup (100g) self-rising flour
1 tsp baking powder
1 tsp cinnamon
$\frac{1}{3}$ cup (100ml) sunflower oil

FOR THE TOPPING
1 cup (200g) low fat cream cheese
1 tbsp powdered sugar
grated peel of 1 orange
few drops vanilla extract

1 Preheat the oven to 325°F/160°C. Lightly grease a deep, 8in (20cm) deep cake pan and line it with waxed paper.

2 In a large bowl, beat together the cottage cheese, sugar, and eggs. Add the remaining cake ingredients and stir well to combine.

3 Spoon the mixture into the prepared cake pan. Bake for $1\frac{1}{2}$ hours, until golden and firm to the touch.

4 Cool the cake in the pan for a few minutes, then take it out of the pan and complete cooling on a wire rack.

5 Beat together the ingredients for the topping and spread over the top of the cooled cake.

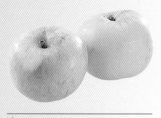

CRUMBLY APRICOT & APPLE BARS

THESE CEREAL AND FRUIT BARS ARE PACKED WITH FLAVOR

AND FIBER. THEY MAKE FILLING SNACKS OR GOOD ADDITIONS

TO LUNCH BOXES.

²/₃ cup (180g) dried apricots
2 tart apples, peeled, cored, and chopped
²/₃ cup (150ml) apple juice
grated peel of 1 orange
1 cup (250g) margarine
¹/₃ cup (75g) light brown sugar, packed
1²/₃ cup (180g) plain whole wheat flour
1 tsp baking powder
1³/₄ cups (200g) rolled oats
¹/₂ cup (60g) chopped nuts

1 Preheat the oven to 350°F/180°C. Lightly grease a 9 x 11in (23 x 28cm) shallow cake pan.

2 Put the apricots and apples in a saucepan with the apple juice and the grated orange peel. Simmer gently for 10 minutes. Cool the mixture slightly and transfer it to a food processor or blender. Process the mixture until smooth.

3 Beat together the margarine and sugar in a large bowl, then fold in the flour, baking powder, oats, and nuts.

4 Spoon half the oat mixture into the prepared pan. Spoon the apricot mixture over the oat mixture and smooth it out. Crumble the remaining oat mixture over the top and press it down lightly.

5 Bake for 30 minutes, until golden. Cut the cake into 16 bars in the pan. Cool on a wire rack before removing the bars from the pan.

★ STAR INGREDIENT
Although any variety of apple is acceptable in this recipe, the best choice is a crisp, tart apple such as Jonathan apples or Granny Smiths.

EACH BAR PROVIDES:

○ Calories 260

○ Protein 4g

○ Carbohydrate 28g
　Fiber 3g

○ Total Fat 15g
　Saturated Fat 3g

○ Sodium 124mg

SERVING TIP
These bars do not need to be eaten as soon as they are baked. Stored in an airtight container, they will keep for up to a week.

Preparation Time: 50 minutes
Makes: 16

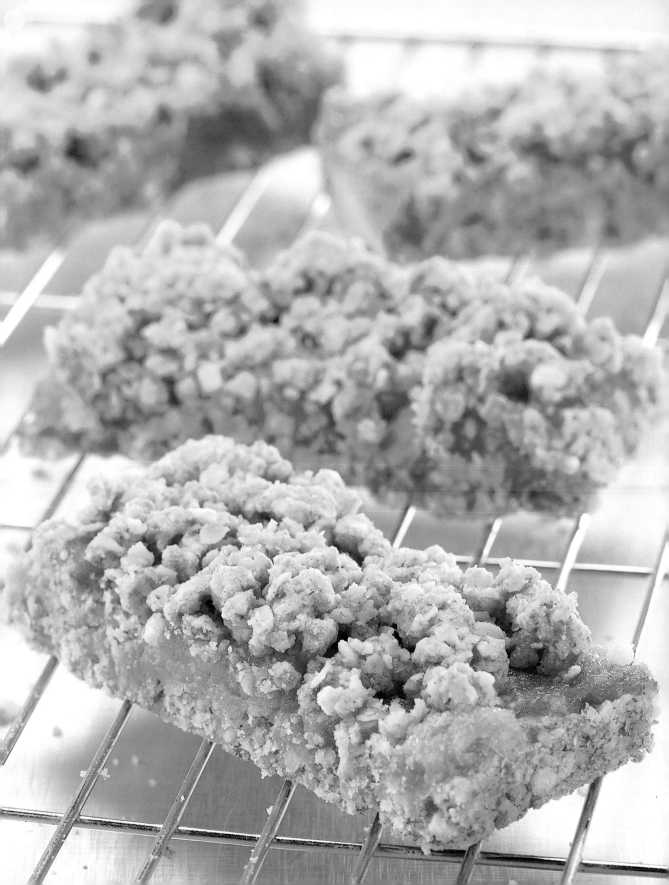

CHOCOLATE BROWNIES

CHOCOLATE BROWNIES ARE A FAVORITE EVERYWHERE.

THIS RECIPE CONTAINS LESS FAT THAN MORE TRADITIONAL

VERSIONS, BUT RETAINS ALL THE FLAVOR.

*8oz (250g) semisweet chocolate,
broken into pieces*
¹/₂ cup (75g) pitted dates
6 tbsp water
1 tbsp baking powder
¹/₂ tsp baking soda
¹/₃ cup (75g) dark brown sugar, packed
1 egg, beaten
1¹/₄ cups (150g) self-rising flour
3 tbsp skim milk
¹/₂ cup (60g) pecans or walnuts, chopped

1 Preheat the oven to 350°F/180°C. Grease a 9in square (23cm) shallow baking pan and line it with waxed paper.

2 Put the chocolate pieces in a heatproof bowl set over a saucepan of simmering water and let the chocolate melt.

3 Put the dates and water in a small saucepan and simmer gently, stirring, until they form a purée.

4 Put the melted chocolate, date purée, and all the remaining ingredients in a large bowl, and mix together well. Transfer the mixture to the prepared pan. Smooth the surface.

5 Bake for 25–30 minutes, until just firm to the touch. Cut into 16 squares. Let them cool in the pan.

✶ STAR INGREDIENT

Pecans are slightly sweeter than walnuts and make a good substitute for them in recipes. Both types of nuts contain polyunsaturated fatty acids, protein, and fiber.

EACH BROWNIE PROVIDES:

○ Calories 171

○ Protein 3g

○ Carbohydrate 25g
   Fiber 1g

○ Total Fat 7g
   Saturated Fat 3g

○ Sodium 42mg

NUTRITION TIP

The date purée is used here as a replacement for the fat that is used in traditional brownie recipes.

Preparation Time: 40–45 minutes
Makes: 16

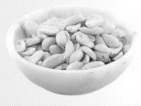

★ STAR INGREDIENT
Unsalted peanuts are available in their shells or shelled. Always check the date: on the package since peanuts quickly lose flavor.

EACH COOKIE PROVIDES:

○ Calories 103

○ Protein 2g

○ Carbohydrate 12g
Fiber 0g

○ Total Fat 5g
Saturated Fat 3g

○ Sodium 40mg

Preparation Time: 20 minutes
Makes: 24

CHOCOLATE PEANUT COOKIES

CHILDREN WILL BE DELIGHTED TO FIND THESE EASY-TO-MAKE COOKIES

IN THEIR LUNCH BOXES. THE COMBINATION OF PEANUTS AND

CHOCOLATE IS IRRESISTIBLE.

$1^2/_3$ *cups (200g) all-purpose flour*
$^1/_2$ tsp baking soda
7 tbsp (100g) unsalted butter
$^1/_3$ cup (75g) dark brown sugar, packed
$^2/_3$ cup (75g) unsalted peanuts,
roughly chopped
2oz (60g) milk chocolate, chopped
1 egg
1 teaspoon vanilla extract

1 Preheat the oven to 350°F/180°C.

2 Sift together the flour and baking soda in a large bowl. Rub the butter into the flour with your fingertips until the mixture resembles fine breadcrumbs. Stir in the sugar, peanuts, and chocolate.

3 Lightly beat together the egg and vanilla and add to the mixture in the bowl. Mix the ingredients together to make a firm dough.

4 Put 24 spoonfuls of the dough on a lightly floured baking sheet, pressing down on each one with the back of a fork. Bake for 10–12 minutes, or until pale golden. Cool the cookies on a wire rack.

INDEX

Page numbers in **bold italics** indicate illustrations. Page numbers followed by an asterisk (*) indicate star ingredients.